DATE DUE

MAY 1 9 1998			
GAYLORD			PRINTED IN U.S.A.

To Renew Books
PHONE (510) 258-2233

Culture, Ethnicity, and Personal Relationship Processes

Stanley O. Gaines, Jr.
with
Raymond Buriel
James H. Liu
Diana I. Ríos

ROUTLEDGE
New York London

Published in 1997 by

Routledge
29 West 35th Street
New York, NY 10001

Published in Great Britain by

Routledge
11 New Fetter Lane
London EC4P 4EE

Copyright © 1997 by Routledge, Inc.

Printed in the United States of America on acid-free paper.

Library of Congress Cataloging-in-Publication Data

Culture, ethnicity, and personal relationship processes /
  Stanley O. Gaines, Jr.
      p.   cm.
    ISBN 0-415-91652-6 (cloth). — ISBN 0-415-91653-4 (pbk.)
    1. Man-woman relationships—United States.   2. Ethnicity—United
States.   3. Intercultural communication—United States.
4. Interpersonal relations—United States.   I. Gaines, Stanley O.,
1961–
HQ801.A2C85   1997   96-49048
306.7—dc21   CIP

Table of Contents

1

Culture, Ethnicity, and Personal Relationship Processes: An Introduction

In a special edition of *Journal of Social Issues* devoted to gender and personal relationships, Winstead and Derlega (1993) declared, "We are born into a gender and into relationships." As numerous reviews (e.g., T. L. Huston & Geis, 1993; Ickes, 1993; Spence, Deaux, & Helmreich, 1985; Wood, 1995) have indicated, the literature on gender-related personality characteristics, gender-role attitudes, and gender *per se* as multi-faceted influences on personal relationship processes is rich and voluminous. The rapid growth of this literature since the early 1970s undoubtedly attests to the impact of the Women's Rights movement of the late 1960s, which in turn owes much of its impetus to the Civil Rights movement of the early 1960s (see Brown, 1986; Spence, et al., 1985).

Few scholars in the field of personal relationships would contest the relevance of gender to academic or lay perceptions of relationship processes (Berscheid, 1994). However, perhaps even fewer scholars in the field seem willing to acknowledge that ethnicity—which, after all, provided the focal point for the Civil Rights movement—also is relevant to the study of personal relationships. Most individuals cannot escape their ethnicity (which many scholars continue to view as equivalent to biological race, especially when considering African Americans; see Landrine & Klonoff, 1996) any more than they can escape their gender (which at least some scholars continue to view as equivalent to biological sex; see French, 1985). Nevertheless, a cursory reading of post-1970s books and articles on personal relationships reveals that ethnicity and related variables (e.g., culture, values) largely have been neglected by personal relationship researchers (Gaines, 1995b).

In this book, my colleagues and I shall examine the ways in which "ethnicity matters" (see West, 1993) as far as genuine understanding of personal relationship processes are concerned. Far from taking for granted the "declining significance of ethnicity" (see Wilson, 1980) vis-à-vis personal relationships, we maintain that culture, values, and ethnicity all are manifested in contemporary relationship contexts in important ways. Moreover, we propose that only by bridging the illusory gaps between the fields of ethnic studies and personal relationships can we as scholars hope to avoid committing the all-too-common "sins of commission" (e.g., falsely assuming that African American or interethnic male-female relationships inherently are dysfunctional); as well as "sins of omission" (e.g., falsely assuming that researchers' witting or unwitting exclusion of Latina/o or Asian American couples from a given sample is tantamount to searching for "culture-free" truths regarding relationship processes) that plague much theorizing and research on personal relationships.

Laying a Foundation for the Study of Personal Relationships: Interpersonal Attraction as Reflected in Interpersonal Resource Exchange

As Heider (1958) observed, personal relationships are integral to the human experience. People have been fascinated by interpersonal relations since time immemorial. As inherently social beings, we want to understand why people interact with each other in a particular manner. As Berscheid (1985) pointed out, human beings are interested especially in understanding the cognitive, affective, and behavioral processes by which people are attracted to each other. Accordingly, some of the most prominent theories within psychology are concerned implicitly or explicitly with the recurring theme of interpersonal attraction.

Berscheid (1985) provided a useful framework for organizing theoretical perspectives on interpersonal attraction. At the most general level, we can identify "social psychological theories that have predictive implications for a number of social phenomena, including attraction" (p. 426). Among social-psychological theories, those that address *reinforcement* (Newcomb, 1956) emphasize the extent to which individuals receive tangible and intangible rewards as a result of interactions with their physical and social environments. Among reinforcement theories, those that address *social exchange* (Homans, 1961) emphasize the extent to which individuals receive tangible and intangible rewards as a result of interactions specifically with their social environments (i.e., with other people). Finally, among social exchange theories, *resource exchange theory* (Foa & Foa, 1974) emphasizes the extent to which individuals specifically receive intangible rewards (i.e., affection and respect) as a result of interactions with other people.

According to Foa and Foa (1974), people need to be loved and held in esteem by significant others. Among the "commodities" or resources that significant others may possess, *affection* (i.e., love, or emotional acceptance of another person) and *respect* (i.e., esteem, or social acceptance of another person) are highly valued. Affectionate behaviors from relationship partners can bolster individuals' self-love, and respectful behaviors from relationship partners can bolster individuals' self-esteem. With regard to interpersonal attraction, not only do relationship partners' affectionate and respectful behaviors *per se* promote attraction, but the *exchange* of affectionate and/or respectful behaviors between partners also promotes attraction.

Interestingly, Berscheid (1985) relegated resource exchange theory to an "auxiliary" status among theories relevant to interpersonal attraction. However, the importance accorded to the classification and exchange of intangible rewards as sources of interpersonal attraction suggests that resource exchange theory is an exemplar of what Berscheid (1985) described as specific theories "principally addressed to particular varieties of attraction . . . and/or to phenomena commonly believed to be associated with attraction" (p. 426). By applying resource exchange theory to the study of interpersonal attraction, therefore, we may gain important insights

3

into human interactions in general and to personal relationship processes in particular.

So far, we have limited our attention to exchange theory (primarily resource exchange theory) as one major reinforcement approach to studying personal relationship processes. Alternatively, reinforcement approaches such as *equity theory* (Adams, 1963, 1965) and *interdependence theory* (Kelley & Thibaut, 1978; Thibaut & Kelley, 1959) might be just as relevant to the study of culture, ethnicity, and personal relationship processes. In response to such a critique, we contend that the exchange/equity dichotomy is false; exchange theory (including resource exchange theory) *is* a form of equity theory (Brown, 1986). Moreover, although recent applications of interdependence theory (e.g., Henderson, 1996; Lin & Rusbult, 1995) show promise as guides to understanding the impact of culture and ethnicity on personal relationship processes, one of the more comprehensive studies to date regarding culture, ethnicity, and relationship processes (Gaines, Rios, Granrose, Bledsoe, Farris, Page, & Garcia, 1996) represents a direct application of social exchange theory in general and resource exchange theory in particular. For these reasons, then, we chose resource exchange theory as one perspective from which to examine culture and ethnicity as predictors of interpersonal behavior within personal relationships.

A Core Model: Interpersonal Resource Exchange in Heterosexual Romantic Relationships

Throughout this book, my colleagues and I shall adopt the perspective that patterns of interpersonal resource exchange characterize heterosexual romantic relationships. In an empirical study of dating and engaged or married couples, Gaines (1996a) reported that (1) women and men tend to reciprocate affectionate behaviors; (2) women and men tend to reciprocate respectful behaviors; (3) women tend to give affection and respect simultaneously; and (4) men tend to give affection and respect simultaneously. From these elements of behavioral covariance, one can construct a core model of interpersonal resource exchange among heterosexual romantic relationships. The resulting core model is presented in Figure 1.1.

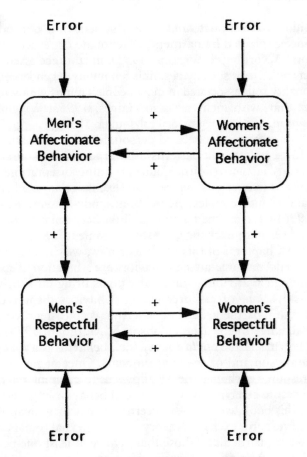

Figure 1.1:
Core model of interpersonal resource exchange

Explicit in the core model of interpersonal resource exchange is the assumption that individuals' resource-giving behavior is influenced largely by their partners' resource-giving behavior. A more implicit assumption concerning the core model is that individuals' resource-giving behavior is *not* necessarily influenced solely or even primarily by their partners' resource-giving behavior. In Gaines's (1996a) study of heterosexual romantic couples, interpersonal traits—especially nurturant or affection-giving traits—explained significant variance in individuals' affectionate *and* respectful behaviors beyond the variance explained by partners' affectionate or respectful behaviors. According to Wiggins (1991), nurturance essentially reflects positive or socially desirable femininity, a gender-related personality trait associated in most people's minds with women rather than with men (see also Gaines, 1995a; Wiggins & Broughton, 1985; Wiggins & Holzmuller, 1978).

Given that gender-related personality characteristics appear to be reflected in patterns of interpersonal resource exchange, is it also true that cultural value orientations are manifested in interpersonal resource exchange among heterosexual romantic couples? At least one study (Gaines, Rios, et al., 1996) has examined empirical links between cultural values and resource exchange; we shall comment further on that study in Chapter 5 of this book. For now, we can assert that individuals' resource-giving behaviors are a function of social-psychological attributes that individuals bring into their relationships *and* of resource-giving behaviors displayed by relationship partners. Such an assertion is consistent with social exchange theory (see Jacobson & Margolin, 1979) and with Lewin's (1936) *field theory* (i.e., behavior is a function of the person and of the environment). Once again, we see that resource exchange theory allows us to examine relationship-specific behavior as well as social behavior in general.

In this book, we will be concerned primarily with applications of resource exchange theory to heterosexual romantic relationships, particularly those that involve at least one person of color. By limiting our focus in this manner, we inevitably invite criticism regarding the external validity of the models presented in this book beyond heterosexual and/or romantic relationships. A study of same-sex and cross-sex friendships by Gaines (1994b), for example, indicated that reciprocity of respect-related behaviors characterizes male-female friendships but not male-male or female-female friendships. In addition, reciprocity of affection-related behaviors does not appear to characterize *any* friendships, whether same-sex or cross-sex in nature. Regarding same-sex romantic relationships, we do not know of any study that has examined interpersonal resource exchange among gay or lesbian couples (see Gaines, 1995b; M. Huston & Schwartz, 1995).

Granted the limitations imposed by our emphasis on heterosexual romantic relationships, we encourage our colleagues in the field of personal relationships to ponder the implications raised by the models of culture, ethnicity, and interpersonal resource exchange presented in this book. In some respects, we have chosen the path of least resistance, given that most theories and research on personal relationships take heterosexual romantic relationships as their point of reference (Berscheid, 1985). In other respects, though, we have departed from the practice of focusing mainly upon Anglo couples that typifies scholarship within the field of personal relationships (Gaines, 1995b; Wood & Duck, 1995). We hope that personal relationship theorists and researchers will consider the plausibility of our conceptual models regarding culture, ethnicity, and interpersonal resource exchange—at least within the circumscribed context of heterosexual romantic relationships—and challenge future researchers to test the limits of applicability of our models.

Culture and Ethnicity as Influences on Personal Relationship Processes

In order to demonstrate the need for a conceptually inclusive, empirically testable account of culture and ethnicity as influences on relationship processes, we must first define key concepts and then document the lack of such an account in current theories and research on personal relationships. *Culture*, according to Ullman (1965), may be defined as "a system of solutions to unlearned problems, as well as of learned problems and their solutions, acquired by members of a recognizable group and shared by them" (p. 5). According to Wilkinson (1993), *ethnicity* refers to "not only a national heritage but also a distinct set of customs, a language system, beliefs and values, indigenous family traditions, and ceremonials" (p. 19). One additional concept that will be crucial to our understanding of the interplay between culture and ethnicity is that of *values*, defined by Smith (1991) as "both features of the world toward which people are oriented and . . . features of people that govern their orientation to the world" (p. 5).

As Reed (1996) has noted, the interplay between culture and ethnicity necessarily is dynamic. That is, the extent to which individuals from a particular ethnic group incorporate the implicit or explicit tenets of a particular culture into their overt and covert behaviors in everyday life may be conceptualized and measured in terms of individuals' internalized value orientations (Braithwaite & Scott, 1991). As such, values are indicative of the transmission of certain aspects of culture into the social-psychological lives of individuals within a given ethnic group. More germane to the present discussion, though, is the notion that cultural value orientations are abstract and of little practical utility in the lives of individuals within a given ethnic group unless they are manifested in social behavior (Gaines, 1995b).

In *Meaningful Relationships: Talking, Sense, and Relating*, Duck (1994) made a compelling case for the importance of culture in the relational lives of individuals. Duck observed that cultural values provide individuals within ethnic groups with particular ways of viewing the world as well as expectations regarding individuals' behavior in a variety of social contexts. This is not to say that all individuals within a specific ethnic group embrace the same cultural values to the same extent. Rather, cultural values give the members of an ethnic group a basis for common ground in terms of overt and covert behavior. Inevitably, however, individual differences in the manifestation of cultural values in interpersonal behavior will arise within an ethnic group.

Individualism and Interpersonal Resource Exchange Among Anglo Couples: An Initial Model of Culture, Ethnicity, and Personal Relationship Processes

In a society as heterogeneous as the United States, it is possible to identify a number of cultural value orientations that individuals from all ethnic groups might incorporate into their thoughts, feelings, and behaviors toward others. However, the tendency for individuals to equate American society with European American culture (Asante, 1994) suggests that some cultural value orientations might be privileged over others. Foremost among value orientations commonly attributed to European American culture is *individualism*, or an orientation toward the welfare of oneself (Gaines, 1995b). Because European Americans constitute the dominant ethnic group in the United States, it might appear that individualism is the only cultural value orientation that Americans embrace. However, individualism is but one of many cultural value orientations that can be found in the rich mosaic of ethnic groups that is the United States (McAdoo, 1993).

Let us assume for a moment that individualism is reflected in patterns of interpersonal resource exchange, at least among Anglo couples. Would we expect an individualistic orientation to promote or deter individuals' displays of affection and respect toward their romantic relationship partners? In the mythology of the United States. individualism is touted as if its positive qualities were self-evident (Bellah, Madsen, W. M. Sullivan, Swidler, & Tipton, 1985). But does a "me orientation" such as individualism really bode well for other-oriented behaviors such as affection and respect? Dion and Dion (1993) concluded that "self-contained individualism" (or, as Bellah et al. [1985] put it, "utilitarian individualism") is *negatively* related to individuals' expressions of trust toward their partners (an important component of affection) and to relinquishing power (an important component of respect; Gaines, 1996a).

The relatively few accounts of individualism and interpersonal behavior that can be found within the personal relationship literature (Bellah et al., 1985; Dion & Dion, 1993) tend to suggest that, contrary to prevailing myths, individualism does *not* promote rewarding relationships, either for highly individualistic persons or for their partners. Instead, individualism seems to promote distrust and power imbalances in personal relationships. These predictions are reflected in an individualistic model of interpersonal resource exchange among Anglo couples, presented in Figure 1.2.

Cultural Values as Multidimensional Influences on Personal Relationship Processes

Given the above discussion of culture and ethnicity, it is clear from various reviews of the available literature (e.g., Bellah et al., 1985; Dion & Dion, 1993; Gaines, 1995b) that one cultural value (i.e., individualism) and one group (i.e., Americans of European descent) have received a disproportionate share of personal relationship researchers' attention. But what about those values that reflect a "we" rather than a "me" orientation? And what about those groups lumped

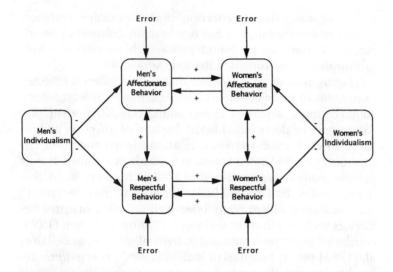

Figure 1.2:
Individualistic model of interpersonal resource exchange among Anglo couples

together under the term "persons of color"? What might we learn from studying cultural values in addition to individualism, and ethnic minority groups in addition to European Americans, that potentially could help us understand relationship dynamics better than we have in the past?

According to Triandis (1990), "non-Western" cultures tend to be characterized not by an orientation toward the success of the individual, but by an orientation toward a larger community. Triandis referred to the "we orientation" involving entire ethnic groups (or, conceivably, involving all of humanity) as *collectivism* (see Gaines, 1994a, 1995b). Triandis (1990) argued that, even in contrast to their counterparts on the continent of Europe (and certainly in contrast to African, Latin, and Asian American cultures), European American culture often de-emphasizes the welfare of the community in favor of the welfare of the individual. Several accounts of collectivism (e.g., Asante, 1981; Gaines, 1994a, 1995b; Hopson & Hopson, 1995), in contrast, indicate that a community-minded orientation is particularly prominent among Americans of African descent.

Even though Triandis's (1990) distinction between collectivism and individualism is useful for our purposes, some aspects of his concepts remain problematic. Consider Triandis's assumption that individualism and collectivism are correlated negatively and strongly (i.e., the more one embraces individualism, the less one embraces collectivism and vice versa). Although Triandis (1990) noted that collectivistic persons can be found within individualistic cultures and individualistic persons within collectivistic cultures, he did not allow for the possibility that a given woman or man might embrace collectivism *and* individualism at the same time.

Recently, Triandis and his colleagues (Gelfand, Triandis, & Chan, 1996) acknowledged that individualism and collectivism might reflect value orientations that essentially are unrelated to each other. Nevertheless, they still have not distinguished clearly between collectivism and another "we" orientation, specifically *familism* (which reflects an orientation toward the welfare of one's immediate and extended family; Gaines, 1995b). In fact, Triandis and his colleagues (Triandis, McCusker, Betancourt, Iwao, Leung, Salazar, Setiadi, Sinha, Touzard, & Zaliski, 1993) went so far as to state that "collectivism across cultures is equivalent to familism" (p. 381, italics removed). Several accounts of familism (e.g., Blea, 1992; Gaines, 1995b; Marin & Marin, 1991; Mirande, 1977) indicate that a family-minded (as distinct from community-minded) orientation is pronounced especially among Latinas/os.

Another "we-oriented" cultural value that may be manifested in personal relationship processes is *spiritualism* (i.e., an orientation toward the welfare of all living entities, both natural and supernatural). Western social scientists generally have shunned spiritualism in their theories and research, apparently out of concern that their work otherwise would be regarded as "unscientific" (Paloutzian & Kirkpatrick, 1995). Particularly as evident in Eastern religions and embraced by Americans of Asian descent (Cook & Kono, 1977; Min, 1995; O'Brien & Fugita, 1991; Tamura, 1994), spiritualism may be a key factor in understanding individuals' interpersonal behavior.

Still another "we orientation" that might be reflected in relationship processes is *romanticism* (i.e., an orientation toward the welfare of one's romantic relationship; Gaines, Rios, et al., 1996). In the social science literature, romanticism often

11

is regarded as identical to individualism (see Bellah et al., 1985; Dion & Dion, 1993). Particularly with regard to interethnic romantic relationships, though, romanticism may be essential to understanding how some couples are able to defy the odds against their long-term success (Gaines, Rios, et al., 1996; Porterfield, 1978; Rosenblatt, Karis, & Powell, 1995).

An Overview of This Book

In the chapters that follow, my colleagues and I begin by examining cultural value orientations that frequently are associated with specific ethnic groups within the field of ethnic studies. First, we consider collectivism as a potential influence on interpersonal resource exchange among African Americans (Chapter 2). Next, we explore familism as a potential influence on interpersonal resource exchange among Latinas and Latinos (Chapter 3). Subsequently, we discuss spiritualism as a potential influence on interpersonal resource exchange among Asian Americans (Chapter 4). Afterward, we look into romanticism as a potential influence on interpersonal resource exchange among interethnic couples (Chapter 5). Finally, we combine the elements of the models from Chapters 1 through 5 into an inclusive model of interpersonal resource exchange, designed to apply to *all* couples (Chapter 6).

Throughout this book, my colleagues and I emphasize that in order for close-relationship researchers to transcend ethnicity conceptually and empirically, they must acknowledge ethnicity in the first place (Gaines, 1995b; Gaines & Reed, 1994, 1995; Reed, 1996; see also Moghaddan, 1987; Phinney, 1996). Thus, we invite you to join us as we mark the trees en route to surveying the forest. In due time we hope that you will challenge us just as we intend to challenge you in this shared intellectual endeavor.

Portions of this chapter were presented by the author during a colloquium at Pomona College, February 22, 1994. Preparation of this chapter was made possible by a postdoctural fellowship from the Ford Foundation (1996–97) and by institutional funds from Pomona College. The author is indebted to Philip Rappaport, two anonymous reviewers, and Steve Duck for their comments on an earlier draft.

2

Collectivism and Personal Relationship Processsess Among African American Couples

In 1977, Alex Haley's best-selling novel *Roots*, published the year before, was adapted for television as an ambitious mini-series. Despite critics' contention that the mini-series was excessively melodramatic (and despite complaints from the Ku Klux Klan that White Southerners were depicted virtually without exception as bigots), this "saga of an American family"—specifically, Alex Haley's own, African American family—became a landmark television event. In an ironic triumph, the concluding episode of *Roots* surpassed the ultimate tribute to the antebellum South, *Gone With the Wind*, to become the most-watched program in television history (Guerrero, 1993). Crucial to the success of *Roots* was its emphasis on the resilience of African and African American personal relationships in the face of unrelenting racism.

In attempting to explain the unexpected and unprecedented success of *Roots*, many critics pointed to the mini-series' articulation of universal themes such as the human longing for a sense of heritage. Indeed, the surge of interest in genealogy (the process by which Haley combed library archives on birth, death, and marriage records, along with slave auction advertisements and news accounts, to trace his lineage back to a village in West Africa) among Whites and Blacks alike seemed to support such an explanation. However, critics tended to discount the impact of a simple yet profound message that *Roots* conveyed: African Americans possess a history and a culture that is theirs uniquely. That is, an unwavering belief in "we-oriented" values reinforced by history and promoted by culture helped sustain personal relationships as African Americans sought to ensure that their biological and fictive progeny would survive despite the tremendous odds against them.

In both Africa and America, Black culture has emphasized a value known as *collectivism*—a value manifested in individuals as a basic orientation toward the welfare of the community. As Triandis (1990) observed, "In collectivist cultures social behavior is determined largely by goals shared with some collective, and if there is a conflict between personal and group goals, it is considered socially desirable to place collective goals ahead of personal goals" (p. 42). To be sure, the co-existence of collectivistic values among persons of African heritage in Africa and in the United States can be attributed in part to the common experience of oppression in Africa, slavery in America, and colonialism with its attendant racism on both sides of the Atlantic Ocean (Gaines, 1996b).

This is not to say that all persons of African heritage embrace collectivism to the same extent, or that collectivism can be found only among persons of African descent. Among African Americans, individual differences in a community-based "we orientation" are evident (White & Parham, 1990), and collectivism can be found among at least some members of all ethnic groups (Triandis, 1990). The primary point here is that the post-1960s literature on African American marital and family relationships frequently cites collectivism as a key to understanding African Americans' personal relationship processes (Gaines, 1994a, 1995b). As such, I will begin by examining collectivism as a potential influence on African Americans' social-psychological lives in general; in turn, I will consider the potential impact of collectivism on African Americans' personal relationships in particular.

Collectivism Among African Americans

At the dawn of the twentieth century, African American leaders such as Booker T. Washington and W.E.B. Du Bois

14

debated the relative importance of economic forces and of cultural values in the eventual empowerment of all African Americans (Gaines & Reed, 1994, 1995). Washington believed that only after African Americans achieved economic self-sufficiency would European Americans grant them social equality. In contrast, Du Bois believed that African Americans' internalization of abstract ideals, such as ingroup pride and social justice, could spur African Americans to transform society so as to redistribute material goods in a more equitable manner among the citizens of the United States. By the middle of the twentieth century, though, Washington's faith in free enterprise *per se* proved to be ill-founded, whereas Du Bois's faith in the power of words and ideas not only had spawned the National Association for the Advancement of Colored People, but had succeeded in striking down government-enforced segregation (Marable, 1986).

In the initial *Handbook of Social Psychology*, Herskovits (1935) contended that "Africanisms" among Blacks in the United States were much more resilient in the face of the physical, psychological, political, and economic assaults of slavery and segregation than had been acknowledged commonly by social scientists and laypersons alike. Despite the fact that African Americans sold into slavery were stripped of the most fundamental human rights and bought, sold, beaten, and even bred like cattle, persons of African descent never relinquished the system of cultural values that they brought to the United States. Drawing in part upon Du Bois, Herskovitz argued that "While in all cases it is the tangible aspects of culture that have been the first to be sacrificed, it is the intangible ones which have persisted most strongly and longest" (1935, p. 261).

Central to African and African American culture is an emphasis on placing the needs of the community (broadly defined) above the needs of oneself. According to Skinner (1987), collectivism as a primary cultural norm has been manifested among persons of African descent since the era of the Atlantic slave trade. Skinner identified the historical periods in which cooperation flourished between and among Africans and African Americans as follows: (1) the "Age of Discovery," characterized by slave revolts; (2) the "abolitionist period," characterized by the struggle for emancipation and by efforts at emigrating from the United States to Africa;

15

(3) the "pan-African phase," characterized by the development of increasingly intricate networks between Africans and African descendants; and (4) the "contemporary phase," characterized by the transition from colonial to autonomous rule among African and Caribbean nations and by greater use of international communications systems (pp. 15–16).

Common to all four historical eras described by Skinner is the phenomenon of self-sacrifice for the sake of the entire Black "race." The cultural message that is evident throughout the various historical eras is that individual success lacks meaning unless it can be used as a tool for helping all persons of African heritage to succeed (White & Parham, 1990). The Rev. Dr. Martin Luther King, Jr. espoused this collectivistic value when, in accepting the 1964 Nobel Peace Prize, he proclaimed the prize a testament to the determination of African Americans to seek equality through nonviolent protest, *and* he used the "world's stage" to condemn apartheid in South Africa (see Gaines, Roberts, & Baumann, 1993).

Given that African American male-female relationships are the foundation for creating families and thus socializing subsequent generations of African Americans regarding cultural values (see Billingsley, 1968), how is a collectivistic orientation expressed in African Americans' personal relationships? In everyday social interactions, African Americans frequently display levels of openness and ease with each other that are not expected or observed in the majority of encounters between African Americans and European Americans (Chimezie, 1984). To the extent that (a) the "me orientation" of individualism is predominant in European American culture and (b) the "we orientation" of collectivism is predominant in African American culture (White & Parham, 1990), we might explain the formality of European American social relationships and the contrasting informality of African American social relationships in terms of the differing cultural value influences operating among the two ethnic groups.

Even though class conflicts do arise among some African Americans, what distinguishes many members of the African American middle class from their European American counterparts is the sense of responsibility cited by the former toward less fortunate members of their ethnic group (Blackwell, 1985). In his theory of the Talented Tenth, Du Bois (1986) gave voice to the cultural norm encouraging African American professionals to work on behalf of the entire ethnic group. Though Du Bois refrained from casting inordinate blame upon the Black middle class for failing to attend to the socioeconomic needs of the Black lower class, Du Bois did caution the middle class against ignoring or neglecting members of the lower class.

Of course, ethnicity and class covary such that European Americans are overrepresented at the upper end and African Americans are overrepresented at the lower end of the socioeconomic spectrum (Boston, 1985). Wilson's (1980) treatise on "the declining significance of race" notwithstanding, interactions *between* European and African Americans generally are characterized by considerable power differentials favoring European Americans (Ickes, 1984). One outcome of those power differentials, at the levels of interpersonal as well as mediated communication, is that African Americans might develop individualistic as well as collectivistic tendencies due to exposure to European American culture (Jones, 1987). However, European Americans are *not* likely to add collectivistic tendencies to their otherwise individualistic repertoire.

Since the late 1960s, several personality scales measuring pro-Black, anti-Black, pro-White, and anti-White dispositions have been introduced to the Black psychology literature (for reviews, see Azibo, 1989; Jenkins, 1995). One such scale, Milliones's (1980) Developmental Inventory of Black Consciousness (DIB-C), classifies individuals according to the following scheme: (1) *Preconscious* (anti-Black and pro-White); (2) *Confrontation* (pro-Black and strongly anti-White), (3) *Internalization* (pro-Black and weakly anti-White), and (4) *Integration* (pro-Black but not at all anti-White; essentially a humanitarian orientation). Implicit in the design of the DIB-C and similar instruments is the assumption that "normal" personality development among African Americans follows a specific sequence, such that individuals must reject negative stereotypes concerning Black culture (and, at the same time, positive stereotypes concerning White culture) before they can appreciate the strengths of their culture (as well as the shortcomings of White culture). Furthermore, such a classification scheme implies that at any given time, all African Americans from adolescence onward can be described by one of the four trait terms (Parham & Helms, 1981).

17

Despite the conceptual promise offered by African American personality scales, it is not clear whether any of those scales actually allows researchers to predict collectivistic (or, for that matter, individualistic) behavior with any accuracy. In fact, what aspects of behavior *would* be predicted by those scales is unclear. Just as mainstream (i.e., European American) personality research has tended to focus on individuals' self-conceptions *per se* rather than on the correspondence between individuals' self-conceptions and overt behavior (Snyder & Ickes, 1985), so too has African American personality research emphasized classification of self-conceptions over the *manifestation* of self-conceptions in individuals' behavior (Sellers, 1993).

Ultimately, whether Blacks progress through a particular developmental sequence en route to a collectivistic orientation in life may be less important to Black-oriented researchers than is the need to place African Americans' personalities *and resulting behavior* within the proper sociocultural context (see Wyne, White, & Coop, 1974). This means that the personality characteristics of, and social behavior among, African Americans cannot be understood adequately when the only frame of reference available is a European American norm for personality and social behavior. Since the bulk of social-psychological research on "ethnicity" seldom considers African Americans *except as social stimuli to whom European Americans are asked to respond*, all too often African Americans are presented as targets rather than as perceivers (Stephan, 1985). Mainstream social psychology may be well-informed as to the cognitive and emotional reactions of European Americans to within- and between-ethnic encounters, but it cannot claim to understand the cognitive or emotional reactions of *African Americans* to within- or between-ethnic encounters (Gaines & Reed, 1994, 1995).

Nevertheless, social psychology has the potential to make creative contributions to the study of collectivism among African Americans. As Wyne, White, and Coop (1974) indicated, Harry Stack Sullivan's (1953) interpersonal theory of personality "is particularly relevant to the Black American experience and speaks directly to what may be expected in the future" (p. 86; but see also Nobles, 1986). Sullivan, who was a neo-Freudian psychiatrist and who brought a distinctly social-psychological perspective to psychiatry (Hall & Lindzey,

1970), believed that the social context was much more active in shaping individuals' personalities than did Freud, who subscribed to a form of psychic determinism (Schellenberg, 1978). Sullivan proposed that *"personality is the relatively enduring pattern of recurrent interpersonal situations which characterize a human life"* (pp. 110–111; emphasis in the original).

Sullivan's interpersonal theory, in turn, was built largely upon Lewin's (1936) field theory; according to Lewin, individuals' behavior must be considered within the scope of their psychological field (i.e., the assortment of social influences to which individuals respond, as well as the personal qualities that individuals bring to bear upon interpersonal settings). If Lewin and Sullivan were correct, then, attempting to interpret African Americans' behavior out of context inevitably will produce profound oversights and misapplications of irrelevant theories of personality. Wyne, White, and Coop (1974) expressed such concerns:

> Until recently, the black self has been conceptualized almost exclusively in terms of the white self. Most research studies have involved a comparison of the self-concepts of blacks with self-concepts of whites, the implication being that the white self is or ought to be the significant other. It has apparently not crossed the minds of most social scientists that an obvious research topic should be aspects of self-concept within the black personality and within the black community. (p. 86)

Considering the fact that even some of the most heralded works on ethnicity (e.g., Allport's *The Nature of Prejudice* (1954); Pettigrew's *A Profile of the Negro American* (1964)) have described African American culture as but a variant on European American culture, it is apparent that the task of incorporating the concept of collectivism into theory and research on personal relationships will not be easy. Nonetheless, if the collectivistic ideal is as pervasive in African American interactions as Afrocentric scholars suggest (e.g., Asante, 1988; Nobles, 1986; Parham, 1993), it is imperative for scholars within the field of personal relationships to take a closer look at collectivism so as to identify those instances in which African Americans do or do not manifest that cultural value in personal relationships.

19

Thus far, I have presented a sociohistorical perspective on African American culture. Such a perspective rarely is found in mainstream theories or research within the field of personal relationships (Gaines, 1994a, 1995b). Unfortunately, the lack of a sociohistorically grounded perspective makes it difficult to eradicate the negative and inaccurate stereotypes regarding African American male-female relationships (i.e., domineering African American women as maintaining the balance of power over effeminate African American men) that still exist in much of popular culture and academia. In the following two sections, I shall examine these prevailing negative stereotypes in greater detail.

Stereotypes: Effeminate Men

In contrast to Herskovits's (1935) contention that African Americans had been successful in retaining basic beliefs and social norms despite the ravages of slavery, in *The Negro Family in the United States* (1939), E. Franklin Frazier argued that slavery severed any cultural ties that transplanted Africans might otherwise have maintained. In order to put Frazier's views in their appropriate sociohistorical perspective, it is important to realize that Frazier was attempting to refute the claim that African Americans were happy under slavery (White & Parham, 1990). However, the message that sociologists and other social scientists tended to extract from Frazier's treatise centered on the alleged "dysfunctionality" of the Black family as a consequence of slavery. Although Frazier had committed precisely those errors against which Herskovits had warned (e.g., characterizing African culture as simplistic, minimizing the perseverance of African values in African Americans), Frazier's work was embraced by mainstream sociology and, ultimately, hailed as a classic (see Hill, 1957).

In keeping with conventional beliefs of that era regarding gender roles, Frazier saw the homes of both European Americans and indigenous Africans as patriarchal in orientation. According to Frazier, however, slaves in America lost autonomy over their preferred mode of familial organization. Also, Frazier surmised, slave families assumed two primary forms: Those families that were acknowledged by European American masters and, thus, influenced by prevailing Anglo social mores were patriarchal, whereas those families that were not allowed to remain intact were bound together through the sheer will of slave mothers, and so were matriarchal.

Upon emancipation, Frazier believed, African American men were more likely than not to turn to lives of vagrancy and sexual recklessness. African American women, on the other hand, were cast as the remaining pillars of strength for their children. These stereotypical views—that is, of the un-reliable Black male and the domineering Black female—were not only accepted by Frazier but were taken at face value by subsequent writers over the ensuing three decades (Gutman, 1976). Though Frazier did not describe African American men as "feminine" per se, many social scientists have inter-preted Frazier's writings as supporting the notion that to the extent that African American men were unreliable, they also were dependent and submissive—in short, effeminate.

The caricature of effeminacy suggests that African Amer-ican men are inept at fulfilling the traditional role of husband/ father as wage earner, subordinate to European American men *and* to African American women, and generally retard-ing the progress of African Americans as a whole (Porterfield, 1978). Such an unflattering portrait of African American men can be understood as cause and consequence of negative im-ages that traditionally have been transmitted by popular me-dia (Spigner, 1992). The image of the African American man as easily intimidated or frightened pervaded newspaper, tele-vision, film, and radio features well into the second half of the twentieth century. Implied by the portrayal of Black men as effeminate, of course, is an underlying opinion of "feminin-ity" itself as undesirable. In any event, the contrast between stereotypes concerning African American men (e.g., as lazy, submissive, and dependent) and those concerning European American men (e.g., as ambitious, dominant, and indepen-dent) is enormous.

With respect to environmental factors that influence African American men's social behavior, a large body of liter-ature has developed around the theme of poverty and the "Black underclass." Much of the substance of President Lyn-don Johnson's War on Poverty program was stimulated by Frazier's (1939) writings on the effects of slavery and eman-cipation upon African American families (C. Williams, 1991). By the late 1960s, a national controversy had erupted over

21

the tacit assumption, reflected in both academic and lay pub-lications (though not necessarily in public policy; see Bianchi & Farley, 1979), that the "Negro problem" lay in the structure of the African American family and that the solution called for carving out a patriarchal niche for African American fathers similar to that enjoyed by European American fathers. Judging by the sociopolitical and academic environment of that time, it appears that (a) many scientific and lay observers equated family and career status with manhood and (b) those same observers equated the high father-absentee and unemployment rates of Black men with lack of manhood.

Despite the reservations that they may have had regarding some of the motives behind the War on Poverty program, many liberals applauded President Johnson (as well as slain President John F. Kennedy) for having committed the federal government to activism in civil rights for disadvantaged persons. Many conservatives, on the other hand, felt that the U.S. government had "gone too far" in helping African American men and their families (Gibbs, 1988). During the post-Civil Rights era, with the exception of the Carter Administration, the federal government has tended to scale back its participation in the reconstruction of American society. Ironically, popular stereotypes concerning the African American man as ineffectual may be more strongly entrenched today than was the case before the 1960s (see Staples, 1977; Taylor, 1977; Wilkinson, 1977).

Afrocentric appraisals of the plight of African American men (e.g., Asante, 1988; White & Parham, 1990) point toward a depiction radically different from that of the "emasculated Black male." As far as the impact of society is concerned, institutional racism (e.g., in penal, educational, and welfare systems) is much more pervasive than either conservatives or liberals have realized (Gary, 1981). As for the "femininity" of African American men, Hall (1981) contended that expressivity is precisely what Black men need—from their families and within themselves—in order to combat institutional racism:

> The family is where the Black male obtains his initial exposure to an environment of support, love, and affection. It is here that he begins to learn about his basic feelings of belonging and trust. If he is able to show fragility in the light of oppressing odds or occasional doubt about what he

should do, and receives support from this intimate inner circle, he will learn to trust the opinions and guidance of those involved with him even after this early stage of life has passed. He can learn and feel how he is to behave when faced with criticism and ascertain from those close to him a validation of his identity and what he as a person is worth to them. He can be dependent upon and nurtured by this support system and assisted in making the choices that will bring about a full life. (p. 161)

By the same token, studies on African American families have paid relatively little attention to the degree to which strong, positive male role models are present in the lives of many young Black males. Not only are two-parent African American families prevalent to a far greater extent than has been acknowledged by most social scientists (Glick, 1988); but even in those situations where the father does not live with the family, an extensive social network composed of uncles, ministers, adult male friends, and other African American men may provide young Black men with many sources of strength and support (Schultz, 1977; Sudarkasa, 1993; Tinney, 1981). All in all, "emasculation" is the exception, not the rule, among African American men.

Some Afrocentrists (e.g., Asante, 1988) have argued that gay Black men represent an affront to Black masculinity. Unfortunately, such a stance equates sexual preference with gender identity (see Brown, 1986). As critics of this homophobic brand of Afrocentrism point out (e.g., hooks, 1992), the error of confusing sexuality with societally prescribed notions of appropriate "male" and "female" behaviors traditionally has been one of the defining features of Eurocentrism. In any event, one can subscribe to the Afrocentric goal of eradicating negative stereotypes of Black men in general without resorting to negative stereotypes of gay Black men in particular.

Perhaps the most dramatic refutation of the "Black male effeminacy" stereotype in recent years was the Million Man March organized by Minister Louis Farrakhan on October 16, 1995 (Karenga, 1995). Although the march was billed as a "Day of Atonement," many African American men viewed the march as nothing less than affirmation that they were worthy of affection and respect in the eyes of society (Boyd, 1995). Despite concerns that misogynist or homophobic themes would emerge in the procession of speeches culminating in Farrakhan's address, such concerns proved to be ill-founded (R. Allen, 1995). The remarkable strength and vulnerability, unity and heterogeneity displayed by approximately one million African American men in Washington, D.C., in front of a global audience (thanks to cable news juggernaut CNN) laid to rest—if only for one day—the notion that Black men inherently are weak or ineffectual (E. Allen, 1995).

So far, I have discussed the myths and realities of Black male social behavior in detail. But what are the myths and realities surrounding the social behavior of African American women? The stereotype of the domineering African American woman stands as the antithesis to that of the effeminate African American man. The reality of African American womanhood, on the other hand, is in many ways similar to that of African American manhood (though key differences must be acknowledged as well). In the next section, I shall consider the theme of the "Black matriarchy" in popular culture and in academia.

Stereotypes: Domineering Women

At the heart of Frazier's (1939) *The Negro Family in the United States* is the claim that African American women emerged through slavery and Reconstruction as the primary authority figures in the African American family. As we noted earlier, Frazier's aim was not to denigrate Blacks but to challenge scholarly and lay misconceptions about African Americans as a group. Nevertheless, Frazier (1939) lent an aura of academic legitimacy to the stereotype that Black women are bossy and domineering toward Black men. The message that many social scientists extracted from Frazier's work can be summarized as follows: African American women are in complete charge of their families, regardless of whether the fathers of their children are present or absent (Porterfield, 1978). Clearly, Frazier did not portray Black women as excessively demanding or forceful (Staples, 1971); yet the myth of the Black matriarchy can be traced largely to subsequent authors' incorporation of Frazier's proclamations into their own scholarly works (Johnson, 1988).

In referring to the "myth of Black matriarchy," I do not mean to imply that female-headed households in themselves are "bad" or that, conversely, male-headed households are "good" (see J. L. McAdoo, 1993). Rather, I am referring to the erroneous belief that female-headed households among African American families are prevalent because African American women inherently are so overbearing as to drive African American men away (Wilkinson, 1993). This mistaken belief obscures the fact that lack of economic opportunity, *not* the supposedly maladaptive personalities or behavior of African American women, poses the biggest obstacle to African American men who would like to meet their obligations as full-time husbands and fathers (Bowman, 1993).

Curiously, the same social-scientific literature that has cast African American women as "pillars of strength" for their families also has cast African American women as psychologically unhealthy. For example, Parker and Kleiner (1966) concluded that Black women were so authoritarian as to have snuffed out any ambitious achievement strivings in their offspring. Even more ominous was the assertion by Parker and Kleiner that no amount of redress of socioeconomic injustices would be sufficient to compensate for the social-psychological damage inflicted by single mothers upon their daughters and, especially, upon their sons.

In response to the claim that single African American mothers somehow stifle achievement motivation in their children, Kriesberg (1967) reported, "Husbandless mothers are generally *more*, rather than less, concerned about the educational achievement of their children, compared to married mothers" (p. 288, italics added). It is the relative lack of support from schools and other agents within communities, *not* presumed psychological shortcomings of Black women, that accounts for the difficulties that single African American mothers face in attempting to encourage their offspring to achieve. In fact, teachers' low expectations of young Black children often counteract single African American mothers' efforts to motivate their children to achieve (H. P. McAdoo, 1986).

Depictions of African American women as unfeminine and/or as co-conspirators (with European American men) in the emasculation of African American men fail to do justice to the extent to which Black women have been victimized throughout their history in the United States (hooks, 1981). Furthermore, the literature promoting the myth of the Black matriarchy is plagued with a variety of double standards concerning African American women. These double standards include: (1) the characterization of female-headed households among African Americans as maladaptive and of female-headed households among European Americans as adaptive (hooks, 1981); (2) the characterization of African American, female-headed households as dysfunctional and of female-headed households among various ethnic groups across the globe as functional (Staples, 1972); and (3) the characterization of female-headed families among African Americans as unnatural and of male-headed families among African Americans as natural (Lammermeier, 1973). Finally, the mass media have tended to accept these and other unflattering comparisons of African American women vis-à-vis persons belonging to other gender/ethnicity groupings (hooks, 1981; Morton, 1991).

One popular myth has it that because of the relatively high rate of out-of-wedlock births among African American females, many African American families (1) have lax sexual standards (especially on the part of Black females) and (2) are responsible for their own poverty (C. Williams, 1991). Yet both lower-class and middle-class African American families wish to provide greater levels of education to their daughters on the matter of contraception (see Fischer, Beasley, & Harter, 1968), and (unlike European American families) single motherhood among African Americans often represents a move, not from self-sufficiency to poverty, but from two-parent to one-parent poverty (i.e., the poverty is present regardless of the marital status of young Black mothers; see Geschwender & Carroll-Seguin, 1990). Like so many other stereotyped beliefs regarding African American women, the myths about sexual promiscuity and disdain for would-be husbands are connected intimately with the larger issue of Black female dominance. However, the theoretical and empirical threads binding such myths together are thin at best.

Much of the literature on African American women focuses on one segment of the population (i.e., lower-class, single mothers), ignores the socioeconomic realities facing that segment of the population (i.e., lack of educational opportunities, lack of financial resources), and proceeds to attribute alleged behavioral defects (i.e., hypermasculine, authoritarian) to the entire population (Malveaux, 1988). For most African American women, though, working to provide food and shelter for themselves and their families never has represented an attempt to showcase their "masculinity" *per se*. In truth, single African American mothers often have had little choice (other than joining the welfare rolls, an action that also is frowned upon by European American culture; see C. Williams, 1991) when confronted with the dilemma of satisfying basic human needs.

Even within the context of two-parent homes, African American women have found it necessary to work in order for families to make ends meet (Geschwender & Carroll-Seguin, 1990; Morton, 1991). As even European American men and women increasingly are realizing (Spence, Deaux, & Helmreich, 1985), dual-income work arrangements no longer are a luxury but a necessity in contemporary American life. Thus, those social scientists and laypersons who blame African American women for usurping the jobs and the pride of African American men do not grasp the severity of the socioeconomic circumstances that millions of African American women and men alike face every day.

Several decades ago, W.E.B. Du Bois (1921/1975) drew attention to the courage of resourcefulness of African American women as made manifest throughout slavery and its aftermath. Instead of casting African American women as the "enemy" of African American men, Du Bois viewed the qualities embodied in African American women as essential to the survival of Blacks in the United States: "To no modern race does its women mean so much as to the Negro nor come so near to the fulfillment of its meaning" (1921/1975, p. 172). In contrast to an individualistic interpretation of the struggles of African American women (e.g., "Black women are snatching away the income and prestige that rightfully belong to Black men"), DuBois's collectivistic interpretation emphasized the contributions that African American women (e.g., Harriet Tubman, Sojourner Truth, Rosa Parks) historically have made for the sake of *all* Black people (see Asante, 1988; Hopson & Hopson, 1995).

By no means have I exhausted the possibilities regarding society's destructive portrayals of African Americans (whether female or male). Indeed, it was not my intention to capture every anti-Black stereotype in this chapter. Instead, I focused on those stereotypes that most frequently are invoked in scholarly and popular depictions of Black male-female relationships. In the next section, I will examine the implications of stereotyped and collectivistic frameworks, in that order, for predicting patterns of interpersonal resource exchange among African American male-female relationships.

Theoretical Perspectives on
African American Relationships

Few topics have been as unsettling within the African American community as has the topic of Black male/female relationships (Asante, 1988; Hopson & Hopson, 1995; Parham, 1993; White & Parham, 1990). Although relational difficulties are by no means unique to African Americans, messages emanating from the mass media might convince one that relationships between African American men and women inherently are conflictual, even pathological in nature. Witness the following account of Black male/female relationships offered by Michele Wallace (1979) in *Black Macho and the Myth of the Superwoman*:

> [The African American woman] has made it quite clear that she has no intention of starting a black woman's liberation movement. One would think she was satisfied, yet she is not. The black man has not really kept his part of the bargain they made when she agreed to keep her mouth shut in the sixties. When she stood by silently as he became a "man," she assumed that he would subsequently grant her her long overdue "womanhood," that he would finally glorify and dignify black womanhood just as the white man had done for the white woman. But he did not. He refused her. His involvement with white women was only the most dramatic form that refusal took. He refused her across the board. He refused her because he could not do anything else. He refused her because the assertion of his manhood required something quite different of him. He refused her because it was too late to carbon-copy the traditional white male/female relationships. And he refused her because he felt justified in his anger. He claimed that she had betrayed him. And she believed that, even as she denied it. She too was angry, but paralyzed by the feeling that she had no right to be. (pp. 14–15)

Wallace's book stirred enormous controversy. Although some scholars (e.g., Morton, 1991; Puryear, 1980) praised Wallace for giving voice to the relational problems plaguing African Americans, other scholars (e.g., hooks, 1981; Powell, 1983) denounced Wallace for having written an inflammatory diatribe lacking in substance. To be sure, Wallace did not start the "battle of the sexes" among African Americans; in certain respects, Wallace may be viewed as a messenger. Nonetheless, Wallace frequently relied on negative stereotypes in attempting to bolster her argument (e.g., the "Black mammy" stereotype as the epitome of the domineering African American woman) and implied that European American male/female relationships were to be regarded as the standard against which all other relationships should be compared.

Like many other writers, Wallace accepted the premise that slavery severed all connections between African Americans and their African heritage. Indeed, to the extent that Black men and women experience difficulty in forming and/or maintaining personal relationships, Wallace's depiction may possess "face validity." However, such a depiction ignores the reality of *successful* relationships between African American men and women.

In his historical analysis of pre-World War II African Americans, Gutman (1976) refuted Frazier's (1939) conclusion that African American men were given to indiscriminate searches for fulfillment of their sexual desires and as lacking in those qualities required for marital stability. Gutman's (1976) work indicates that, although African Americans have not had the material resources commonly taken for granted by European Americans, many Black couples and families did in fact possess the *socioemotional* resources needed to sustain personal relationships. All too often, contemporary researchers seem to assume that the amount of material resources available to individuals is proportional to the amount of intangible resources that are available (e.g., Foa and Foa (1974) described the African American community as lacking in both tangible and intangible resources; Gaines, 1994a). One must wonder how African American relationships have been formed and maintained, given such a pessimistic portrayal of those relationships within the social science literature.

In an effort to incorporate collectivistic themes into the understanding of relationship processes among African Amer-

icans, Asante (1981) identified several dimensions of Afrocentrism that might be displayed in personal relationships:

> There are four aspects of Afrocentric relationships: *sacri-
> fice, inspiration, vision,* and *victory.* In each of these as-
> pects, we see elements of mutual respect and sharing. (p.
> 77) From this fountain flows all the good that we do for
> each other and our people. . . . It is an impossibility to be
> one with each other Afrocentrically and not be one with
> the people. The one who claims to love you but does not
> love the people is attempting to deceive you. This occurs
> most often when individuals have deceived themselves into
> believing that they can separate their love for you from
> their love for the people and still remain Afrocentric. This
> is not possible. (p. 81)

Asante contended that (a) collectivistic values sustained
African American couples and their families throughout centuries of slavery, and (b) such values are integral to the future of
all African Americans. Unlike Frazier (1939), who believed that
the "natural" role of African American men (and, in fact, *all*
men) should be that of uncontested heads of households, Asante (1981) described an egalitarian gender-role arrangement
as one that corresponded most clearly with an Afrocentric perspective. Therefore, Asante's analysis indicates that African
American couples' adherence to collectivistic norms actually
would militate against male-oriented gender-role arrangements.

In *Friends, Lovers, and Soul Mates: A Guide to Better
Relationships between Black Men and Women,* African
American clinical psychologists/spouses Derek Hopson and
Darlene Hopson (1995) drew explicitly upon Asante's work
in offering advice to African American couples. Hopson and
Hopson suggested that in order to build a solid socioemotional foundation for their relationships, African American
women and men ideally should (1) take pride in their cultural
heritage, (2) refer to that heritage continually in the process of
defining themselves, and (3) act toward each other in a manner consistent with that heritage. If African American couples
immerse themselves in the collectivistic traditions embraced
by persons of African descent throughout the Diaspora, the
Hopsons believed, partners in African American relationships
will attend thoughtfully to each other's needs for love and es-

teem. Moreover, Hopson and Hopson (1995) contended that by behaving in accordance with collectivistic norms, an African American couple increasingly will view their own relationship as an important source of social and psychological strength for the entire African American community.

White (1984; see also White & Parham, 1990) went so far as to link collectivism with egalitarianism in African American male/female relationships. White observed that, decades before social and personality psychologists acknowledged *en masse* the errors in conceptualization and operationalization of "masculinity" and "femininity" (e.g., the assumption that the two traits were mutually exclusive; the assumption that "masculine" women and "feminine" men were not only psychologically deviant but likely to prefer sexual relations with members of their own gender), ideals that ultimately would be referred to by Bem (1974), Spence (Spence, Helmreich, & Stapp, 1974), and other researchers as "androgynous" were accepted by large portions of the African American community. Moreover, White (1984) argued, African Americans often strove to affirm the dual presence of self-directed and partner-directed qualities in themselves even as European American culture held up caricature-like images of ineffectual men and dominant women as objects of scorn.

I hasten to note that collectivism *in and of itself* does not necessarily predispose African Americans to be egalitarian in theory or in practice. Historical materialists (e.g., Lemelle, 1993; Margolis, 1984) have suggested that, ultimately, egalitarian behavior (or lack thereof) reflects the concrete economic reality of the times—*not* the abstract value orientation of a particular group of people. Out of sheer necessity, African American women always have worked (Spence, Deaux, & Helmreich, 1985). Not coincidentally, socioeconomic forces traditionally have not allowed African American men to become the sole breadwinners within their homes even when they desired such a role (Bowman, 1993). In the absence of explicit data collection and hypothesis testing with regard to the impact of collectivism on African American male-female relationship processes (Gaines, 1994a, 1995b), we must acknowledge the viability of the historical-materialist perspective on African American relationships.

Nevertheless, if Afrocentric theorists such as Asante (1981), Hopson and Hopson (1995), and White (1984; White

31

& Parham, 1990) are correct in their assessments regarding collectivism and egalitarianism, we might expect that African American couples tend to value flexibility in women's and men's roles and behavior (Hill, Billingsley, Engram, Malson, Rubin, Stack, Stewart, & Teele, 1993). Some support for this hypothesis is evident in African American teenagers' perceptions of husband and wife roles as symmetrical (King, 1969). Furthermore, African American men tend to place greater priority upon the ability of their ideal wives to participate in power-sharing relationships than do European American men (see Melton & Thomas, 1976). Moreover, African American husbands tend to share in decision-making processes with their wives rather than make decisions autonomously (Dietrich, 1975; J. L. McAdoo, 1993). Interdependence (as indicative of collectivism) seems to be preferred over independence (as indicative of individualism) as a primary goal of husbands and wives in African American marital relationships.

Now that I have discussed stereotyped and collectivistic perspectives on personal relationship processes among African American couples, let us consider the ways in which these perspectives might be incorporated into the core or "generic" model of interpersonal resource exchange that initially was presented in the previous chapter. Remember that in the generic model (which did not take ethnicity into account), reciprocity of (a) affection and of (b) respect was cast as functional behavior within the context of marital and other romantic male-female relationships. However, based on the stereotyped model described earlier in this chapter, one might expect that any displays of affection or respect by African American women toward African American men will be reciprocated by African American men—but not vice versa. In other words, among African American relationships, the stereotyped model would predict that the influence of women's behavior on men's behavior overshadows the influence of men's behavior on women's behavior. The stereotyped model is presented in Figure 2.1.

Now consider the manner in which the collectivistic perspective might inform our original, generic model. According to Asante (1981), men's as well as women's internalization of collectivistic norms will be manifested positively in reciprocal displays of affection and respect among African American

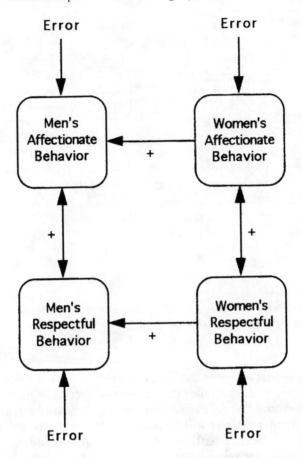

Figure 2.1:
Stereotyped model of interpersonal resource exchange among African American couples

couples. The net effect of the collectivistic model, then, would be to acknowledge that African Americans' affectionate and respectful behavior is not just a function of their partners' behavior but also is a function of a specific value orientation emphasizing oneness with the larger African American community (Gaines, 1994a, 1995b). The collectivistic model is presented in Figure 2.2.

What evidence, if any, can we muster in support of the collectivistic model of African American couples' patterns of

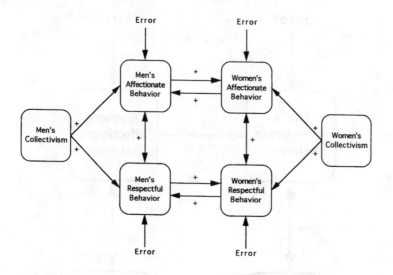

Figure 2.2:
Collectivistic model of interpersonal resource exchange among African American couples

interpersonal resource exchange? In the following section, I shall review those studies that address directly the matter of interpersonal resource exchange among African Americans. Of particular interest will be evidence that collectivism actually does influence patterns of affection-giving and respect-giving behavior among African Americans.

Empirical Research on African American Relationships

Earlier in this chapter, I discussed the utility of Sullivan's (1953) interpersonal theory for the study of interpersonal resource exchange between African American men and women. One aspect of Sullivan's theory dealt exclusively with the process of give-and-take in personal relationships: Sullivan's *theorem of reciprocal emotion.* This theorem represents a significant part of the conceptual foundation for the resource exchange theory that would be developed by Foa and Foa (1974) some twenty years later. Sullivan applied the theorem of reciprocal emotion directly to the topic of interpersonal behavior:

> *Integration in an interpersonal situation is a reciprocal process in which (1) complementary needs are resolved, or aggravated; (2) reciprocal patterns of activity are developed, or disintegrated; and (3) foresight of satisfaction, or rebuff, of similar needs is facilitated.* (p. 199, emphasis in original)
>
> So far as the positive aspect of this theorem manifests itself, complementary needs are resolved in the interpersonal relations one lives through; reciprocal patterns of activity are developed, refined, made more perfect; and there is foresight of how satisfaction can be gained more quickly, or continued longer, by improved performance. (p. 199)

Though Sullivan did not articulate the content of interpersonal behavior (Carson, 1969), it is obvious that, at least from the perspective of resource theory (Foa & Foa, 1974), affection and respect are reciprocated on a regular basis in mutually satisfactory personal relationships. To the extent that African American men and women follow collectivistic norms (Asante, 1981), they are likely to engage in such adaptive forms of resource exchange (Hopson & Hopson, 1995).

Drawing upon Sullivan's (1953) views on interpersonal intimacy, Comer-Edwards (1988) suggested that the achievement of high levels of intimacy *in the face of daunting socioeconomic obstacles* could provide African American couples with the resolve needed to bring about individual-level and couple-level satisfaction. According to Comer-Edwards, intimacy in affectionate and respectful behavior among African American couples may be prevalent especially among middle-class Blacks, who presumably have surmounted many, if not most, of the societal barriers that have kept many of their lower-class brothers and sisters generally frustrated and, at times, angry in their individual and social lives.

Comer-Edwards's (1988) interpretation of social class as a potent influence on intimacy and interpersonal resource exchange between African American men and women may aid in interpreting the finding (Triandis, Weldon, and Feldman, 1972) that lower- and working-class Black women often displayed greater levels of disrespect for Black men than did middle-class Black women. Perhaps some African American women in the lower socioeconomic echelons of society, who often are single mothers and consequently are at tremendous risk for poverty (French, 1985), have been stymied so frequently and so severely in their attempts at securing individual and relational happiness that they have become jaded—justifiably so—when it comes to potential romantic relationships with African American men. To date, however, such an account has not been verified empirically.

Ironically, empirical studies on African American male-female relationships have cast resource exchange primarily in terms of money and other tangible resources, rather than those intangible resources over which African Americans historically have had the most control—love and esteem. With regard to kin networks, H. P. McAdoo (1978), Savage, Adair, and Friedman (1978), Hoffereth (1984), Gaudin and Davis (1985), Zollar (1985), and Taylor (1986) all operationalized interpersonal resource exchange in terms of money. Regarding male-female relationships specifically, Staples (1985) went so far as to contend that marital lifestyles and marital stability among African Americans were governed by individuals' (and, typically, men's) socioeconomic worth. In so doing, Staples explicitly rejected the view (e.g., Darity & Myers, 1984) that African American women were stymied in their search for lifelong partners by the relatively low numbers of African American men, in favor of the view that the *quality* of Black men (again, mostly with regard to level of education and/or income) was so low, on average, as to be detrimental to traditional family structure.

Staples (1985) did not consider the possibility that, despite their historical and contemporary lack of access to tangible resources, African Americans never relinquished their hold on affection or respect as interpersonal resources. Even Foa and Foa (1974), whose resource theory represented a clear break with the mainstream view among exchange theorists that interpersonal behavior was dictated by zero-sum gain motives (Berscheid, 1985), nonetheless focused upon Blacks' relative inability to secure tangible resources in everyday life (Gaines, 1994a). Thus, it is not surprising that very little research has been directed toward reciprocity of affectionate or respectful behavior among African Americans' heterosexual romantic relationships.

Some studies (e.g., Gray-Little, 1982; for a review, see Willie & Greenblatt, 1978) have addressed power and decision-making processes in African American families, but few studies have indicated that marital or family researchers understand that marital roles do not, in and of themselves, convey meaningful information about African American partners' socioemotional behavior. Even fewer studies actually have included a discussion of collectivism along with affection-giving or respect-giving behaviors among African American couples. Triandis, Weldon, and Feldman (1972) conducted one of the small number of studies concerning collectivism and interpersonal resource exchange among Blacks; it is to this study that I now turn.

According to Triandis, Weldon, and Feldman (1972), "There is . . . a stronger tendency to *admire* [i.e., show respect toward], and *love* [i.e., show affection toward] ingroup members in the black data, when compared with the white" (p. 83). Among African Americans, men were more likely to lend assistance to, go out socially with, and show respect toward women than were other women. Moreover, African American women were more likely to go out with African American men than were other African American men. However, it was not clear whether African American women actually reciprocated lending of assistance or displaying respect toward African American men.

It seems, then, that the potential for high levels of exchange regarding affectionate and respectful behaviors among African American couples is substantial. Unfortunately, the aforementioned suppositions about African American male-female relationships typically have not been verified empirically within the context of actual personal relationships. Triandis, Weldon, and Feldman (1972) did not ask individuals to comment on the extent to which they displayed affection or respect toward specific heterosexual partners. Instead, respondents were asked to indicate the extent to which they tended to engage in a variety of behaviors toward African American men and African American women *en masse*. Triandis's work, therefore, provides us with tantalizingly relevant data but with little evidence as to what really happens in African American male-female relationships.

Future research based upon Triandis's (1990; Triandis, Weldon, & Feldman, 1972) work on collectivism and interpersonal resource exchange among African Americans might compare the impact of individualistic and collectivistic norms upon affectionate and respectful behavior in Black male-female relationships. For instance, in an empirical study, Bell, Bouie, and Baldwin (1990) reported that African American men and women who adopted a collectivistic orientation were more likely to display affection-giving and respect-giving behavior toward Blacks of the opposite gender than were African American men or women who adopted an individualistic orientation (though the scenarios to which participants responded were hypothetical in nature). Though Bell, Bouie, and Baldwin did not deal specifically with interpersonal resource exchange, their results indicate that individualistic norms inhibit reciprocity of affection and respect, whereas collectivistic norms facilitate such reciprocity, among African American couples.

But what about those African American marriages that stand the test of time? Is it within those marriages that collectivism is most strongly evident? Clearly, Triandis's work on affectionate and respectful behavior among African and European Americans can aid researchers in forming hypotheses as to the prevalence of collectivistic ideals among specific Black couples. All things considered, though, social scientists interested in interpersonal resource exchange among African American couples should examine reciprocity using the couple as the unit of analysis.

Summary and Conclusions

In considering African American marital relationships and collectivism, I am reminded that many practitioners and academicians, Black as well as White, believe that the distinctions that can be made between Black and White cultures are few and relatively minor. For instance, in *The Nature of Prejudice*, Allport (1954) stated that Black culture and White culture were virtually indistinguishable. Although Allport's (1954) treatise is regarded as a classic to this day (and rightfully so, given its scholarly refutation of racist ideology in science and in the "real world"), even Allport did not attempt to identify "Africanisms" in African American culture as a whole (Gaines & Reed, 1994, 1995). Also, as I mentioned earlier, Frazier (1939) argued against racist interpretations of the Black family, only to fall prey to biases and errors himself.

Throughout this chapter, I have alluded to the promise offered by a collectivistic model in yielding a portrait of interpersonal resource exchange among African American couples that is not just "more sympathetic" than one would expect from most pre-Civil Rights era treatments of Black male-female relationships. Ideally, the collectivistic model should explain significantly greater variance in African American women's and men's interpersonal behavior than does a stereotyped model. My primary challenge has been to provide an account that is at once retrospective and prospective, that rediscovers African Americans' pre-slavery history and places contemporary African American personal relationships within a broad temporal context. I believe that the task of taking scholarship on African American socioemotional behavior "back to the future" barely has begun, however. I am hopeful that in time a growing body of empirical research comparing the relative merits of the "stereotypical" and "collectivistic" models of reciprocity in affectionate and respectful behavior among Black couples will accumulate within the personal relationship literature.

Preparation of this chapter was made possible by a postdoctoral fellowship from Franklin and Marshall College (1991–92), by a postdoctoral fellowship from the University of North Carolina at Chapel Hill (1992–93), by a postdoctoral fellowship from the Ford Foundation (1996–97), and by institutional funds from Pomona College to Stanley Gaines. The author expresses gratitude to Steve Duck, Bernadette Gray-Little, Philip Rappaport, two anonymous reviewers, and especially Sheila Walker for their comments on an earlier version of this chapter.

3

Familism and Personal Relationship Processes Among Latina/Latino Couples

Stanley O. Gaines, Jr., Diana I. Ríos, and Raymond Buriel

In decades past, a book on culture, ethnicity, and personal relationship processes likely would have been confined to theories and research on African Americans, because of the assumption that "Black" and "minority" somehow are interchangeable terms (see Moore & Pachon, 1985; A. Ramirez, 1977). However, as we approach the twenty-first century in the United States, the fallacy of this assumption is all too apparent. Both Blacks and Whites have been slow to recognize the rapid growth and influence of a broadly defined ethnic group that at one time laid claim to one-third of what now is the continental United States. As has been the case with African Americans, Latinas/os can lay claim to a unique history and culture, displaying considerable tenacity while simultaneously responding to changes in Anglo culture over time (Buriel, 1984; Moore & Pachon, 1985; M. Ramirez, 1983; Rios, 1993; Sanchez, 1993; Williams, 1990). Through this process of acculturation, ethnic minorities in general (Harrison, Wilson, Pine, Chan, & Buriel, 1995) and Latinas/os in particular (Buriel & Saenz, 1980) may become bicultural as an adaptive response to the dual influences of majority and minority cultures.

Most African Americans were born in the United States, trace their roots to the American South, and identify not so much with a particular African nation as with the entire continent of Africa. In contrast, the diverse array of individuals who are classified as Latinas/os or Hispanics (at least by Anglos, if not by themselves; Bean & Tienda, 1988; Buriel & Cardoza, 1988; Moore & Pachon, 1985) are separated within the United States both by current geographic locales and by national origins. Specifically, Mexican Americans (i.e., Chicanas/os) are represented primarily in the Southwestern states (primarily California, Texas, and New Mexico), Cuban Americans in Florida, and Puerto Ricans in New York (Moore & Pachon, 1985).

Acknowledging the diversity in group identifications and regional settlement patterns among the nation's Latinas/os, what (if any) core values can be said to characterize Latina/o culture? In the preceding chapter, we noted that a dominant cultural theme within African American psychology is that of collectivism (i.e., an orientation toward the welfare of one's community, broadly defined). Within Latina/o psychology, however, a somewhat different cultural theme emerges. Many authors (e.g., Hurtado, Rodriguez, Gurin, & Beals, 1993; Marin, 1993; Mirande, 1977; Moore & Pachon, 1985; Sanchez, 1993; but see also Bean & Tienda, 1988) have pointed to *familism*, which Marin and Marin (1991) defined as "a cultural value that involves individuals' strong identification with and attachment to their nuclear and extended families, and strong feelings of loyalty, reciprocity, and solidarity among members of the same family" (p.13) that transcends national and regional affiliations among Latinas/os. Consequently, in this chapter, we explore the ways in which individuals' orientation toward the welfare of their immediate and extended family (as distinct from an orientation toward the welfare of individuals' larger communities; Cabrera, 1971; Gaines, 1995b) affects the course of personal relationship processes in general and interpersonal resource exchange in particular.

Familism Among Latinas and Latinos

Based on the social-scientific literature on Latinas/os' cultural values, it appears that familism has been a defining feature of Latinas/os throughout their history in the United

States (Mirande, 1977). The results of some studies indicate that *la familia* (a term that encompasses extended as well as immediate family; Mirande, 1977; Sena-Rivera, 1979) is not as central to the lives of many Latinas/os as was the case in previous decades (Suarez, 1993; Willems, 1975; Williams, 1990). Nevertheless, empirical studies continue to suggest that familism is more pronounced as a cultural value among Latinas/os than among Anglos (Marin, 1993; Mindel, 1980) or among African Americans (Mindel, 1980). Moreover, familism appears to form part of the basis for cultural common ground among Mexican Americans, Puerto Ricans, Cuban Americans, and other Latina/o groups (Dieppa & Montiel, 1978).

We do not mean to imply that familism can be found only among Latinas/os, or that familism is unrelated to any other cultural value. Familism is evident among members of all ethnic groups to some degree (see Bean & Tienda, 1988). Furthermore, familism is correlated positively with collectivism as a "we orientation" (Gaines, Marelich, et al., 1996; see also Triandis, 1990). Nevertheless, Latinas' and Latinos' orientation toward their immediate and extended families has been cited in a variety of studies as an influence on Latinas/os' interpersonal behavior (Chilman, 1993; Mirande & Enriquez, 1979; Sanchez, 1993).

When it functions at its best, the family does not command allegiance but engenders loyalty through its nurturance and ability to adapt to individual (as well as societal) change (Abalos, 1986). In Latina/o families, it is common for parents, relatives, and ceremonial kin or *compadres* to devote considerable attention to the socioemotional needs of children (Harrison et al., 1995; Schmidt & A. M. Padilla, 1983; Sjostrom, 1988). In turn, children often display a high degree of respect toward their elders (Kephart & Jedlicka, 1988; Paz, 1993). These patterns of reciprocity between older and younger family members frequently are passed along from one generation to the next, even when family networks are disrupted by relocation (e.g., from Mexico to the United States).

In order to gain a better understanding of the impact that familism has upon the everyday lives of Latinas/os, it is important to understand the degree to which members of this diverse group have struggled to maintain a sense of cultural identity (Cabrera, 1971; Meier & Ribera, 1993; Mirande,

1977; Moore & Pachon, 1985; Rios, 1993; Sanchez, 1993). Consider the experiences of *Mexican Americans*, who comprise the majority of the population of Latinas/os in the United States (i.e., roughly 60%; Bean & Tienda, 1988). Until the middle of the nineteenth century, Mexico owned virtually all of the territory that today is known as the southwestern portion of the United States (see Mirande, 1977). However, in the 1850s, relations between the United States and Mexico changed dramatically.

Most of what formerly had been Mexican territory was sold to the United States. Thus, Mexican Americans originally did not become American through immigration. Mexican Americans were, in fact, Mexicans who became American by virtue of military rule. As such, Mexican Americans were subjected to *internal colonialism* by the United States (Blauner, 1972). Since that time, Mexican Americans (i.e., Chicanas/os) have fought to retain their cultural heritage in the face of overwhelming societal pressure toward assimilation.

Like Mexican Americans, *Puerto Ricans* (the second-largest Latino group in the United States, or approximately 14%; Bean & Tienda, 1987) have retained a rich cultural heritage largely through sheer effort. In the fifty years since Operation Bootstrap was established in Puerto Rico by U.S. entrepreneurs, Puerto Rico has been transformed into a virtual colony of the United States (Samoiloff, 1984). Because of the unusual financial and diplomatic relationship between the two countries, persons born in Puerto Rico are considered citizens of both Puerto Rico and the United States.

For many Puerto Ricans, dual citizenship has been a mixed blessing at best; in both countries, Puerto Ricans have become the poorest of all Latina/o groups (Rodriguez, 1992). It is a testimony to the efforts of Puerto Rican and Mexican American families that both groups have survived despite the socioeconomic obstacles befalling them (see Carroll, 1975; Schaefer, 1988). In fact, Latinas/os in general earn lower wages than do either Anglos or African Americans (Chilman, 1993; French, 1985).

In contrast, *Cuban Americans* (the United States's third-largest Latino group, constituting about 6%; Bean & Tienda, 1987) have not had to deal with poverty, unemployment, or other negative consequences of prejudice and discrimination to the same extent as have Mexican Americans or Puerto

Ricans. The financial assistance lent by the United States government to the initial wave of Cuban expatriates, the wealth that many of those expatriates brought with them to the United States, and the overwhelmingly White phenotype of the early Cuban refugees all contributed significantly to the relatively advantaged status that Cubanas/os *en masse* have enjoyed (Bean & Tienda, 1988; Chilman, 1993; Moore & Pachon, 1985; Suarez, 1993). Nevertheless, like other Latina/o groups, many Cubanas/os have found it necessary to guard themselves against societal pressures toward cultural as well as structural assimilation (Gernard, 1988).

To what degree do Latinas/os experience conflict between embracing the familistic norms espoused by their own culture and embracing the individualistic norms espoused by Anglo culture? The answer to such a question may depend upon whether Latinas/os themselves are allowed to respond, or whether members of the dominant majority respond "on behalf" of Latinas/os (see Rios, 1994). From the vantage point of Latinas/os, it is clear that one can pursue goals that are prized by Anglo culture (e.g., individualism) while remaining committed to the norm of familism (see Garza & Lipton, 1984; Rueschenberg & Buriel, 1989). Just as one may become fluent in the languages of both cultures, so too may one become fluent in the values of both cultures (i.e., bicultural/multicultural; see Ballesteros, 1979; Buriel & Saenz, 1980; Harrison et al., 1995; Moore & Pachon, 1985; Paredes, 1993; Ramirez, 1984; Rios, 1993; Sanchez, 1993).

This is not to say that one can understand Latinas/os and their culture simply by superimposing a familistic model of personality and interpersonal behavior over an already existing (i.e., Anglo-oriented) individualistic model. Acosta (1984) noted that concepts such as "success" may be interpreted differently by Latinas/os and Anglos. For many Latinas/os, the "me-oriented" strivings characteristic of Anglo culture are but of secondary importance when compared with the desires to uphold the family name, to send money back to *la familia* out of a sense of conviction rather than guilt—in other words, the "we-oriented" strivings that are essential to maintenance of a familistic ethic. As Dieppa and Montiel (1978) put it, many members of Latina/o cultures routinely reconcile potentially conflicting individualistic and familistic norms by supporting a "commitment to individual autonomy *within the context of familial and traditional Hispanic values*" (p. 5, italics added).

For many Latinas/os, familism and individualism need not be seen as mutually exclusive sets of values. Thus, the problem is not one of deciding which set of values is "better," but rather one of pursuing both goals when the majority culture rejects familism and stresses individualism instead (see Menchaca, 1989). A similar theme of duality in collectivistic and individualistic strivings in the context of a predominantly individualistic society has characterized much of the social science literature on African Americans from W.E.B. Du Bois onward (Du Bois, 1903/1969; see also Gaines & Reed, 1994, 1995; Jenkins, 1995; Jones, 1987; White, 1984; White & Parham, 1990).

Ironically, when mainstream social scientists *have* detected traces of individualism in Latina/o culture, they have tended to infer that the culture itself is dysfunctional (Paredes, 1993). Nowhere is this tendency within the social science literature more apparent than in discussions regarding so-called "machismo" within Latino culture (Vasquez, 1994; Wilkinson, 1993). In the next two sections, we shall discuss stereotyped assumptions regarding Latinos' hypermasculinity and, correspondingly, Latinas' hyperfemininity as evident in mainstream treatises on Latinas/os and familism.

Stereotypes: Macho Men

In European and European American culture, priority is placed upon individual strivings (Bellah et al., 1985; Triandis, 1990). Some forty years before the modern Women's Rights movement, Adler (1927/1968) argued that individualism in Anglo culture is manifested in male-oriented prejudice and discrimination:

> As a consequence of the development of culture in the direction of personal power, especially through the efforts of certain individuals and certain classes of society, who wish to secure privileges for themselves, this division of labor has fallen into characteristic channels which have colored our entire civilization. The importance of the male in the culture of today is greatly emphasized as a result. The division of labor is such that the privileged group, men, are guaranteed certain

advantages, and this as a result of their domination over women in the division of labor. Thus the dominant male assures advantages and directs the activity of women to the end that the more agreeable forms of life shall appertain always to the males, whereas those activities are allowed women which men can advantageously avoid. (p. 103)

In many respects, Adler's words ring as true today as they did during the 1920s. Margolis's (1984) account of gender roles in the United States from colonial times to the latter half of the twentieth century bears witness to Adler's assertions. As Margolis pointed out, some American psychologists have stood out historically as chief protagonists of male privilege. For instance, John B. Watson is regarded widely as the father of American behaviorism; it is not as widely known, however, that Watson frequently authored popular-media articles in which he cautioned women to appreciate the grave importance of their role as mothers, as trainers of future presidents (and, we might imagine, presidents' wives). At any rate, it is apparent that tremendous inequities favoring males have been part and parcel of American culture in decades past, just as it is apparent that such inequities are not likely to disappear in the foreseeable future.

A review of the literature on Anglo and Latina/o cultures, however, reveals that social scientists typically have described Anglo cultures as egalitarian and Latina/o cultures as male-oriented *when comparing the two cultures* (Zinn & Eitzen, 1987). Consider Ellis's (1971) characterization of Latina/o and Anglo folkways:

Latin America is dominated by the male. It has been said that Latin America is man's country, and to a large extent this is true. *Machismo* is not only a virtue but a way of life. Familial life is strongly patriarchal and introspective. . . . The woman's place is in the home; the daughter is to be sheltered, protected, and chaperoned. For the Latin American, the North American family is much too liberal, too undisciplined, and ineffectual in influencing the lives of its members. (p. 172)

In Ellis's account, several features of the predictably stereotyped portrayal of Latina/o culture are evident: (1) the emphasis on *machismo* (i.e., exaggerated sense of masculinity; see Lucero-Trujillo, 1980) ostensibly as the primary norm operating in Latina/o culture; (2) the corresponding de-emphasis on familism *per se* as a cultural value; (3) the depiction of Latina/o families as fundamentally patriarchal; and (4) the description of Anglo culture as egalitarian in contrast. Aside from the fact that Ellis (1971) failed to acknowledge that Mexico is part of North America, Ellis was successful in incorporating all of these interrelated stereotypes into a seemingly plausible characterization of Latina/o culture. Even more intriguing is the fact that Ellis (1971), like many other writers before and since, presented this characterization as if it were untainted by possible bias or misinformation (Mirande, 1977; Paredes, 1993).

Taken to its extreme, the rationale favoring machismo as the primary Latina/o cultural norm would suggest that when familism and *machismo* clash within a given household, machismo will prevail. This is exactly the view that many social scientists have adopted (e.g., Goldwert, 1980; Penalosa, 1968; Sanchez-Ayendez, 1986). In turn, social scientists frequently associate machismo with Latino psychopathology and with cultural dysfunctionality (e.g., Figueroa-Torres & Pearson, 1979; Goldwert, 1980, 1982; Liebman, 1976; Paredes, 1993).

The "cult of masculinity" associated with Latinos has been accorded a place in many psychoanalysts' jargon as the Don Juan syndrome (e.g., Marmour, 1951; McClelland, 1987; see also G. Lewis, 1963). Even Adler (1927/1968) invoked the imagery of Don Juan, the legendary Spanish conquistador/womanizer, as the prototype of the hypermasculine male (see Ramirez, 1983; but see also Miranda & White, 1993). But what evidence has been mustered by those social scientists adhering to the opinion that such a personality type exists? Moreover, what counterevidence has been marshaled by those researchers who have declared such an account biased as well as flawed?

In case studies such as *Five Families* (1959) and *La Vida* (1963), Oscar Lewis established himself as a key proponent of the "cult of masculinity" perspective as well as the related concept of the "culture of poverty." Curiously, in *Five Families* (1959), Lewis believed that his study of five predominantly lower-class Mexican families would help dispel many myths about the lower classes in general and about Mexican lower classes in particular. Lewis credited himself with having used the family, rather than the individual, as the unit of analysis in his study. However, Lewis's conclusions—which he framed as illustrative of Mexican culture regardless of social class—only served to reinforce prevailing stereotypes.

In *La Vida* (1963), Lewis undertook an intensive study of one Puerto Rican extended family. Lewis felt that *La Vida* represented a methodological advance over *Five Families* in that several biographies now were gathered regarding each individual under investigation. Also, Lewis cautioned social scientists not to make an inordinate number of negative inferences about the family under investigation. Nevertheless, Lewis seemed unaware that in continuing to propagate the view that a "culture of poverty" (i.e., a way of life endemic to Puerto Rico as well as Mexico) somehow caused illegitimacy, drug abuse, and other social problems, he was just as vulnerable to gross misperceptions as were those social scientists who argued that the individuals themselves fundamentally were dysfunctional. In other words, Lewis's cultural determinism was no more accurate than was the Freudians' psychic determinism as a framework for understanding the impact of large-scale socioeconomic factors (e.g., job availability, education, income)—none of which were under the control of the family in Lewis's (1963) study—upon the everyday lives of Latina/o families.

Interestingly, Lewis (1959) offered a tautological description of Mexican men. If they are domineering, Mexican men may be regarded as suffering from psychological disorders (e.g., the Don Juan syndrome). But if they are *not* domineering, Mexican men still may be regarded as suffering from psychological disorders (e.g., impotence). With the pseudo-Freudian hypothesis that Mexican men are maladjusted no matter what the results, one cannot go wrong in "explaining" the behavior of Mexican-origin and other Latino men (see Guthrie & Lonner, 1986).

Based upon Lewis's conclusions, it would seem that if "blame" is to be placed as to Latinos' lower socioeconomic status compared to Anglos (Vasquez, 1984), likely culprits are to include Latina/o culture and/or Latina/o families (see Harrison et al., 1995). The usual explanation is as follows: Latinos place an excessively high emphasis on machismo, thus creating family settings that are unstable and contingent upon the whims of father figures. The unstable family structure, in turn, inhibits children's ability to take advantage of the opportunities afforded them by Anglo culture. Finally, these children grow up having internalized these negative personality traits and display them once they establish their own families.

Part of what makes such explanations puzzling is the fact that Latina/o culture is criticized for having precisely those qualities that many social scientists have deemed favorable in Anglo culture *when comparing Anglo culture to Black culture* (Zinn & Eitzen, 1987). That is, Anglo culture has been praised as promoting the "natural" (i.e., male-dominant) gender-role arrangement, whereas Black culture has been criticized for promoting a supposedly matriarchal social structure (e.g., Clark, 1965; Frazier, 1957). As we shall see shortly, the Anglo-Latino comparison that places Anglos in a favorable light is just as unsubstantiated as is the Anglo-Black comparison that likewise favors Anglos (Staples & Mirande, 1980). For now, however, we wish to stress that both forms of traditional majority-minority comparison are based upon the belief that Anglo culture is "better." Far from reflecting a "value-free" assessment of Latina/o culture, then, conventional scholarship has reflected a negative, value-laden judgment (Paredes, 1993; Ramirez, 1983).

Ramos and Ramos (1979) observed that Latina/o culture frequently is portrayed in the social science literature as "traditional," while Anglo culture is portrayed as "progressive." With regard to *machismo*, such a dichotomous portrayal obscures the fact that American culture tends to promote those values (i.e., individualistic values) stereotypically associated with Anglo men (French, 1985; Paredes, 1993). Moreover, the Anglo-Latino dichotomy presented above fails to acknowledge the fact that *machismo* simply does not define Latina/o culture to the extent that scholars and laypersons alike generally have believed.

Paredes (1993) offered an even more damning critique of the emphasis on *machismo* in mainstream social scientists' description of Latina/o culture. According to Paredes's accounts of Mexican folklore along the Texas-Mexico border, the terms *macho* and *machismo* did not even appear in Mexicanos' or Chicanos' everyday language before World War II!

Apart from the issue of what Anglos and Latinos believe to be the defining characteristics of a "real man," then, we must wonder whether psychoanalytic interpretations of Latinos as suffering from the Don Juan syndrome represent anything more than just another example of the naming fallacy at work (see McClelland, 1987).

Empirical research on Latina/o families conducted since the late 1960s has called into question many widely held beliefs concerning machismo as a predominant cultural norm among Latinos (Chilman, 1993). In particular, contemporary researchers have indicated that (1) familism and machismo constitute conceptually distinct cultural norms, and (2) when the two sets of values come into conflict, familism tends to prevail. In decades past, even those social scientists who were attuned to the problematic nature of much of the research on Latinos often constructed surveys in which questions regarding machismo were included as part of scales purportedly measuring familism (e.g., Diaz-Guerrero, 1984). More contemporary research, however, suggests that familism as a cultural norm explains many behavioral phenomena that simply cannot be explained by machismo.

Davis and Chavez (1985) reported that the support of family and friends helped unemployed husbands/fathers maintain positive self-esteem as well as their identity as men during the times that their wives were providing all of the income for the households. Furthermore, in a review of studies on decision-making processes, Cromwell and Ruiz (1979) surmised that the "cult of masculinity" supposedly determined the nature of marital and family relationships among Latinos was a myth. Also, although Levine and Bartz (1979) reported that Chicano parents were not as equalitarian in their child-rearing attitudes as were Anglos or Blacks, the same authors (Bartz & Levine, 1978) added that Chicano, Anglo, and Black families all were equalitarian. As Mirande (1985) pointed out, the emerging school of thought regarding familism and *machismo*—a school of thought developed primarily by Mexican American social scientists—actively refutes the stereotypes and untested assumptions of the old school.

Commenting on Latino families in Central America, Knight (1979) also observed that the "cult of masculinity" has been misinterpreted in previous research. Knight proposed that the term *dignidad* is more accurate than is *machismo* in capturing the feelings of pride expressed by many Hispanic men (see also Paredes, 1993). Indeed, the attention that many Latino fathers devote to their offspring (Kephart & Jedlicka, 1988) can be understood more readily as a manifestation of paternal pride (e.g., Carrasco, Wilkins-Vigil, & Auslander, 1977) than as a manifestation of male dominance (e.g., Liebman, 1976).

Returning to Adler's (1927/1968) discussion of personality and social behavior, it is interesting to note that Adler viewed affiliative motives as of secondary importance when compared with power-seeking motives as directing personality development. However, Adler (1927/1968) also hinted that familism might take precedence over individualism in those cases where value clashes were imminent: "To have one's own way all the time is possible only within the circle of one's family, and not always there" (p. 165). Moreover, Zapata and Jaramillo (1981) found Adler's interpretation of family interactions compatible with the results of their study on gender roles in Chicana/o families. Not only was a father-bias absent in the roles that offspring attributed to parents, but parents did not display a son-bias in the roles that they attributed to offspring. Moreover, Schmidt and A. M. Padilla (1983) noted that Latina/o grandparents tended not to make strict gender-based distinctions when interacting with grandchildren. Overall, *la familia* does not conform very well to the "cult of masculinity" that frequently is presumed to pervade Latina/o culture (Marin & Marin, 1991).

As for the "Don Juan syndrome," perhaps Freud fancied himself a conquistador (Goldwert, 1980), but little evidence exists that most Latino men perceive themselves as such. Much has been written about the "Latin lover" from a psychoanalytic perspective (e.g., G. Lewis, 1963; Hayner, 1954; Liebman, 1976; Pierson, 1954; see Marmour, 1951; McClelland, 1987), but seldom have social scientists paused to consider the contradictions inherent in their portrayals of the "cult of masculinity." How is the Latino husband/father supposed to be able to maintain iron-fisted rule over his family yet remain able to desert his family at a moment's notice? These contradictions persist in much of the social science literature on Latinos because the basis for theorizing vis-à-vis *machismo* lies in mythology, not in fact (Mirande, 1977).

As we have seen thus far, the stereotype of the "macho" Latino is overblown. Nevertheless, the stereotype continues to find favor in some academic circles. In addition, a complementary stereotype concerning the "submissive" Latina has surfaced in much of the social science literature. It is to this latter stereotype—and the evidence against it—that we now turn.

Stereotypes: Submissive Women

If machismo represents the stereotype of exaggerated masculinity among Latinos, then *marianismo* may be viewed as the stereotype of exaggerated femininity among Latinas (Goldwert, 1980; Sanchez-Ayendez, 1986; Stevens, 1973). In contrast to the *macho* who supposedly is compelled to assert his sexuality whenever possible (before as well as after marriage), according to much of the social science literature, the *mariana* is depicted as virtually asexual, as interested primarily in motherhood but not in the act that produces motherhood. Furthermore, the stereotype holds, Latinas are so obedient as to be childlike (Chilman, 1993; see also Moore & Pachon, 1985). Although marianismo (also labeled *hembrismo* by some social scientists; Moore & Pachon, 1985) as a concept might seem especially outdated in this post-Civil Rights, post-Women's Rights era, in some respects that stereotype seems even more firmly entrenched in social scientists' minds than does machismo.

The "cult of femininity" stereotype regarding Latinas stands in sharp contrast to the "cult of matriarchy" stereotype regarding African American women described in the previous chapter (see also Gaines, 1995b). Many writers have assumed that widespread rape of African American women by European American men during slavery left African American women embittered and hostile toward men in general (and African American men in particular), whereas widespread rape of Native American women by European American men during colonization left Native American women and, consequently, *mestizas* conquered and submissive toward all men, and toward Latino men in particular (for examples, see Frazier, 1939; Goldwert, 1982; Hernton, 1965; Liebman, 1976). Exactly how such divergent stereotypes of Latinas and of African American women evolved is unclear.

The divergence in stereotypes is so great that one must wonder how either stereotype—whether of the submissive Latina
or of the domineering African American woman—can be
taken at face value.

Whatever the origins of the stereotype concerning the
"cult of marianismo," the stereotype appears routinely in the
social science literature. Consider the following passage from
Goldwert (1980):

> Underpinning male-female relations in Mexico and Spanish
> America is the widely accepted assumption of the superiority
> (biological, intellectual, and social) of the male. Although she
> is sometimes placed on a pedestal, especially in courting
> time, the female is less valued than the male. Because she is
> ambivalently rejected by male-oriented culture, the female
> tends to identify with the children. This she is able to do be-
> cause she had already assumed feminine identification with
> her own self-denying and submissive mother, an outcome of
> the close mother-daughter relationship. (p. 49)

According to such an account, the only substantive relationships in Latina/o culture are those between mothers and
offspring (especially daughters). Furthermore, the Latina is
portrayed as reactive rather than active in shaping her own
destiny. Moreover, Goldwert's (1980) account suggests that
Latinas are quite willing to lead married lives fraught with
subjugation just so that they can experience the short-lived
euphoria that presumably results from courtship. Goldwert's
description of Latinas and marriage is similar to that provided by McGinn (1966) but differs somewhat from that of
Gonzales (1986), who places greater emphasis on the benefits
that Latinas derive from motherhood in and of itself. However, Goldwert (1980), McGinn (1966), and Gonzales (1986)
all indicate that the question for Latinas is not whether they
will become mothers but whether they will do so *within the
context of marriage*, and not whether they will give birth but
how often they will give birth (see also Espin, 1986).

This is not to say that either virginity or motherhood *per se*
should be viewed as tantamount to Latina oppression (Aamott
& Matthaei, 1991). In fact, both values may be viewed as consistent with familism (Gonzales, 1986) and with basic tenets of
Catholicism (Espin, 1986). Rather, we are attempting to call at-

tention to the degree to which Latinas' *choice* regarding virginity and/or motherhood has been ignored in much of the available literature (Bean & Tienda, 1988; Chilman, 1993). Again, at issue is the belief—whether expressed explicitly or implicitly—that Latinas are incapable of making their own decisions in everyday life (Gonzales, 1979).

Even those scholars who hope to promote greater awareness of interpersonal relations involving Latinas sometimes reinforce negative stereotypes about Latinas. Ironically, so do some researchers whose evidence refutes the myth of the submissive Latina (Mirande & Enriquez, 1979). With the advent of the modern Women's Rights movement in the United States, several scholars (e.g., Kiram, Green, & Valencia-Weber, 1982; Liebman, 1976; Mayo, 1978; Soto & Shaver, 1982; Tharp, Meadow, Lennhoff, & Satterfield, 1968) have begun to challenge the notion that Latinas see themselves as inferior to their husbands or fathers. However, many of those scholars have concluded that Latinas are just beginning to assert themselves *in response to American egalitarianism*. The possibility that Latinas have laid claim to their rights and to their own identities, both in historical and in contemporary times, is rarely entertained by social scientists.

That so many scholars point toward the "liberalizing" influence of the United States upon Latino culture is odd, considering the extent to which Latinas and Latinos alike have felt exploited in the name of "American interests" in Latin American countries as well as in the United States (Acura, 1988). In any event, a growing body of research now indicates that (1) the "cult of marianismo" is overstated and that (2) Latina activism was not invented by European American feminists. For instance, in South America, Radcliffe (1990) and Corcoran-Nantes (1990) have observed the distinction between the worlds of politics (associated with men) and of *la familia* (associated with women) never have been as isolated from each other as has been the case historically in European/European American countries. Moreover, whatever self-determining efforts currently are undertaken by Latinas represent but the latest in a series of sociopolitical moves dating back at least to the turn of the century (Burns, 1982).

Now that we have explored the stereotypes that continue to dominate much discourse on Latinas and Latinos, we shall consider the "mini-theories" that would be derived from stereotyped and familistic conceptualizations of Latina/Latino relationships. In the following section, we will present two competing models of Latina/o relationship processes: (1) a model that takes heterosexual romantic relationships "out of context" (i.e., a stereotyped model of interpersonal resource exchange) and (2) a model that places such relationships firmly within such a context (i.e., a familistic model of interpersonal resource exchange). The stereotyped model of Latina/o resource exchange represents a degradation of the original Foa and Foa (1974) model, whereas the familistic model represents an elaboration of the original Foa and Foa model (see Gaines, 1995b).

Theoretical Perspectives on Latina and Latino Relationships

The results of some studies (e.g., Hartzer & Franco, 1985) suggest that sex-typing occurs with regard to Latinas' and Latinos' performance of household tasks (i.e., husbands take care of relatively infrequent outdoor tasks and wives take care of relatively frequent indoor tasks). However, sex-typing in household task performance is not confined to Latina/o relationships by any means (see Atkinson & Huston, 1984). This is not to excuse androcentrism within Latino *or* Anglo cultures (Vasquez, 1994). We simply wish to point out that even those results that ostensibly point toward gender differences in Latinas' and Latinos' execution of household chores do not necessarily reflect "machismo" or "marianismo" *per se.*

According to Lara-Cantu (1989; Lara-Cantu & Navarro-Arias, 1986), Latinas and Latinos alike are capable of "masculine" and "feminine" traits and behavior. In addition, in an empirical study of personality traits among Chicanas, African American women, and European American women, Zeff (1982) reported, "The results . . . do not support the prevailing view in the literature that describes Mexican American families as patriarchal with Mexican American women [as] feminine, docile, and submissive" (p. 257). Also, in an empirical study of Mexican and Mexican-American farm labor families, Hawkes and Taylor (1975) observed, "Dominance-submission patterns are much less universal than previously assumed or never existed but were an ideal or undergoing radical change" (p. 807). Clearly, a one-dimensional view of Latinas and Latinos is inconsistent with many of the findings generated by contemporary personality theory.

The stereotyped depictions that we have discussed so far would lead one to believe that only two types of Latinos and Latinas exist in the Americas—that is, self-aggrandizing men and self-sacrificing women. However, just as role flexibility is common in African American male-female romantic relationships (as described in the preceding chapter), so too is role flexibility common in Latina/o romantic relationships (Harrison et al., 1995). Blea (1988) elaborated upon the variety of roles available to Latinas and Latinos in real-life marital relationships:

> Women are strong in Chicano culture. They are strong as cultural and decision-making symbols, and they are strong physically. Cultural and historical social conditions have demanded that both males and females work hard. Both men and women value home life. Women are not hesitant to work alongside men in maintaining their home. After working long hours during the week (longer than most white men for the same pay), Chicano men do not hesitate to work around their homes. Increasingly, more men are involved in childrearing. (p. 41)

As Vasquez (1994) observed, mainstream social scientists have maintained assumptions regarding Latino men as exhibiting excessive masculinity and Latinas as exhibiting excessive femininity for several decades with virtually no empirical evidence supporting those assumptions. Perhaps it is no coincidence that the stereotypes of Latinas and Latinos are so different from those that persist of African Americans. After all, if we are to assume that (1) both African American and Latina/o relationships inherently are dysfunctional; *and* (2) African American relationships are reverse sex-typed, unlike "normal" Anglo relationships in which men are dominant over women; *but* (3) Latina/o relationships resemble Anglo relationships in terms of traditional gender role arrangements, the only way for Latina/o relationships to be rendered "abnormal" is for one to assume that any pattern of sex-typing among Latina/o couples must be excessive when compared with that of Anglo relationships. This type of convoluted thinking would help explain why the caricature of Latino men reflects *hyper*masculinity and the caricature of Latinas reflects *hyper*femininity.

If familism is as important to Latinas/os' social lives as research would suggest (Harrison et al., 1995; Marin, 1993; Marin & Marin, 1991, Mirande, 1977), we might expect a familistic orientation to permeate Latinas' and Latinos' marital relationships. Consistent with this prediction, results reported by Hawkes and Taylor (1975) suggest that egalitarian behavior may reflect the influence of familism on the behavior of Latinas and Latinos (see also Harrison et al., 1995). Those results contradict the assumptions of Diaz-Guerrero (1975), who viewed Chicana mothers as controlling affection (but not respect) and Chicano fathers as controlling respect (but not affection) as interpersonal resources within families.

At this juncture, we might examine the divergent predictions that would be made using (a) stereotypic and (b) familistic models of interpersonal resource exchange between Latinas and Latinos. In the stereotyped model, socioemotional behavior is taken "out of context" and is assumed to proceed such that Latino men's displays of affection and respect significantly influence Latinas' displays of affection and respect—but not vice versa. Notice that this stereotyped prediction is exactly opposite to that presented in the previous chapter regarding African American relationship processes. The stereotyped model of interpersonal resource exchange among Latina/o couples is presented in Figure 3.1.

In the familistic model, on the other hand, Latina/o interpersonal resource exchange is placed within the context of familism as a cultural value orientation. In this latter model, familism is assumed to contribute positively to displays of both affection and respect. Furthermore, clear patterns of reciprocity of both affection and respect are assumed to occur among Latina/o couples. The familistic model of interpersonal resource exchange among Latina/o couples is presented in Figure 3.2.

Empirical Research on Latina-Latino Relationships

In this section, we address those studies that specifically have focused upon affection-giving and respect-giving behav-

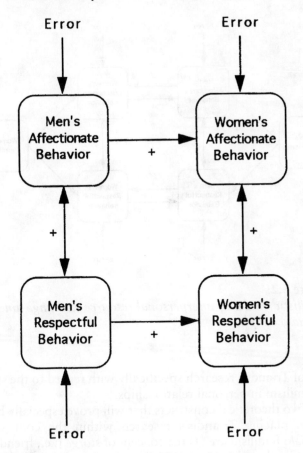

Figure 3.1:
*Stereotyped model of interpersonal resource exchange
among Latina/o couples*

ior among Latinas and Latinos. Virtually the only research
conducted regarding interpersonal resource exchange among
Latinas/os is that of Triandis and his colleagues (e.g., Triandis, Hui, Albert, Leung, Lisansky, Diaz-Loving, Plascencia,
Marin, Betancourt, & Loyola-Cintron, 1984; Triandis,
Marin, Lisansky, & Betancourt, 1984; for reviews, see Marin,
1993; Marin & Marin, 1991; Triandis, 1990). We shall discuss some of Triandis's work on Latinas and Latinos in detail.
In addition, we will comment on the strengths and shortcom-

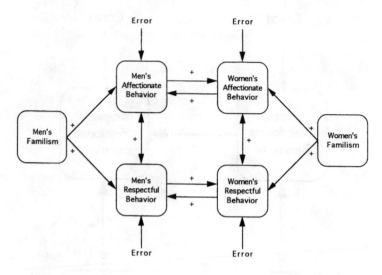

Figure 3.2:
Familistic model of interpersonal resource exchange among Latina/o couples

ings of Triandis' research specifically with regard to the study of familism in personal relationships.

Two theoretical constructs that will prove especially helpful in placing Triandis's research within the context of Latina/o familism are (1) the concept of *storge* (i.e., friendship love) developed by Lee (1976) and subsequently by Duck (1986; see also Fehr, 1993), and (2) the concept of *simpatia* (i.e., an emphasis on harmonious interpersonal behaviors) developed by Marin and Marin (1991; see also Triandis, Marin et al., 1984). We shall examine these relational constructs in greater detail to set the stage for Triandis's work.

Lee (1976) identified six forms of love that partners may experience in personal relationships. One of these, *agape* (i.e., all-giving love) is humanitarian in nature and will not be discussed further. Of the five remaining types of love, Lee distinguished among *eros* (romantic love), *mania* (possessive love), *ludus* (game-playing love), *storge*, and *pragma* (logical love). Subsequently, Duck (1986) described *storge* as the hallmark of those personal relationships that have progressed beyond initial attraction (i.e., beyond romantic, possessive, and game-playing forms of love) and the impetus to partners' decisions regarding permanency in their relationships (i.e., the impetus to pragmatic love).

Marin and Marin (1991) defined *simpatia* as a cultural script among Latinos: "*Simpatia* emphasizes the need for behaviors that promote smooth and pleasant social relationships. As a script, *simpatia* moves the individual to show a certain level of conformity and empathy for the feelings of other people. In addition, a person with *simpatia* ("*simpatico*") behaves with dignity and respect toward others" (p. 12). Although Marin and Marin interpreted *simpatia* as indicative of the influence of *collectivism* rather than familism per se, Triandis' (1990) overview of *simpatia* would imply that the type of "we orientation" reflected in that cultural script is directed toward the family specifically (rather than the more community-based "we-orientation" of collectivism; Gaines, 1995b).

Triandis, Hui, Albert, Leung, Lisansky, Diaz-Loving, Plascencia, Marin, Betancourt, and Loyola-Cintron (1984) reported the results of two studies on idiographic models of interpersonal behavior. In Study 1, 10 social scientists were asked to provide a minimum of 2,400 judgments apiece regarding the likelihood that an actor in a particular culture would engage in each of a series of 20 behaviors across each of a series of 120 interpersonal situations. Each of the 10 social scientists (i.e., Triandis, Hui, Albert, Leung, Lisansky, Diaz-Loving, Plascencia, Marin, Betancourt, and Loyola-Cintron) was familiar with a particular cultural context (7 social scientists had been raised in either U.S. Hispanic or Latin American cultures, 1 had been raised in a European culture, and 2 had been raised in Asian cultures) and limited his or her judgments to that cultural context. Results indicated that Latinos (regardless of nationality) tended to view male-female pairings as higher in friendship than they viewed male-male pairings. The results of Study 1 fit well with Duck's (1986) characterization of "storge" or friendship love—requiring mutual displays of both affection and respect—as an essential prerequisite to success in marriage.

In Study 2, 31 participants (each of whom was familiar with a specific cultural context) from a variety of educational backgrounds were asked to provide 640 judgments apiece regarding the likelihood that an actor would engage in each of a set of 10 behaviors across each of a set of 64 social situations. Of the 31 participants in Study 2, eight had participated in Study 1 as well. Results indicated that a "Mexican factor" emerged among participants such that persons scoring high on the factor "emphasized subordination and friendliness" (p. 1398), whereas persons scoring *low* on the factor viewed gender as a salient discriminating variable and were somewhat hostile as individuals. These results are congruent with the expectation that familism and *machismo* are negatively related (i.e., familism promotes relatively stress-free social interaction and *machismo* promotes stressful interaction among Hispanics).

Triandis, Hui et al. (1984) interpreted the results of both studies as evidence for norms of affectionate and respectful behavior operating among Latinos. Of the two conceptual models (i.e., stereotypical and familistic) that we have identified as possible frameworks for comprehending and anticipating Latina/o interpersonal resource exchange, only the familistic model would have allowed us to predict accurately the impact of high and low scores of the "Mexican factor" on interpersonal dynamics. Especially intriguing was the revelation that in Latina/o culture, persons high in educational accomplishments frequently are expected to display humility when musing on their individual success. However, whether the sample used by Triandis and colleagues was representative of Latinas/os as a whole is not clear (see Harrison et al., 1995).

In a subsequent article, Triandis and his colleagues (Triandis, Marin et al., 1984) reported the results of a study on *simpatia* as a cultural script. Three samples of Latino and non-Latino Navy recruits served as participants in the study. The first sample consisted of 41 Latinos and 49 non-Latinos, each of whom was asked to provide a total of 260 judgments regarding the likelihood that an actor would engage in each of a set of 5 to 11 behaviors across each of a set of 32 interpersonal situations. Also, a subset of the questionnaire items was given to two civilian samples, a group of 60 bilingual college students in the Los Angeles area and a group of 50 monolingual upper-division high school students in Puerto Rico. Triandis, Marin, Lisansky, and Betancourt (1984) found that Latinos were more likely than were non-Latinos to expect displays of affection and respect to occur in social situations.

The second sample consisted of 60 Latinos and 62 non-Latinos, each of whom was asked to provide a total of 600 judgments regarding the likelihood that an actor would engage in each of a series of 20 behaviors across each of a series of 30 role-relationships. Triandis, Marin, Lisansky, and Betancourt (1984) found that Latinos and non-Latinos gave significantly different responses on 47 of the 600 items; although the number of significant responses was far smaller than the number of *nonsignificant* responses, the number of significant differences nonetheless was higher than the number (30) that one would expect by chance. Moreover, 36 of the 47 significant differences were in the expected direction (i.e., *simpatia* was evident to a greater degree among Latinos than among non-Latinos).

The final sample in the Triandis, Marin, Lisansky, and Betancourt (1984) study consisted of 51 Latinos and 54 non-Latinos, each of whom provided the same number of total judgments (600), based on the same number of behaviors (20) and role-relationships (30) as did participants in Sample 2. In Sample 3, Latinos and non-Latinos gave significantly different responses on 117 of the 600 items. Furthermore, 50 of the differences were significant at the .01 level or lower. Of the 50 differences that were significant beyond the .01 level, 38 were in the expected direction (i.e., *simpatia* was evident to a greater degree among Latinos than among non-Latinos). All in all, Triandis, Marin, Lisansky, and Betancourt (1984) concluded, *simpatia* constituted a key value within the rubric of familism among Latinos.

However, Triandis, Marin, Lisansky, and Betancourt (1984) noted several instances of behavior in role-relationships, particularly in the results from Sample 3, that did not fit *simpatia*. Among the unexpected findings was the instance of Latinas/os tending to see husbands as more likely to give orders to their wives than did non-Latinos. Nevertheless, most of the results in the Triandis et al. study supported the "familistic orientation" hypothesis of Latina/o resource exchange.

Taken together, the results reported by Triandis and colleagues are consistent with the prediction that familism facilitates affection-giving and respect-giving behavior in Latina/Latino relationships. Despite the conceptual appeal of Triandis's work, methodological problems limit the extent to which the results can be cited as proof regarding actual relational dynamics. That is, in no instance did Triandis or his colleagues ask participants to assess *their own relationships* with regard to interpersonal resource exchange.

Ironically, Triandis's studies on Latina/Latino relationships have focused upon the *individual* rather than the family or even the dyad as the unit of analysis. Although individual-level data in and of themselves need not be disparaged (McCall & Simmons, 1991), the individual-level data collected by Triandis and colleagues do not speak to the question of participant-as-actor—or, for that matter, participant-as-observer. Instead, participants serve as cultural commentators—again, an important perspective to acknowledge but not to be relied upon exclusively. Unfortunately, the very phenomena that Triandis and colleagues have addressed (e.g., *simpatia*, familism) are rendered abstract and never made concrete.

We do not mean to indict Triandis's research on Latinas and Latinos. Indeed, Triandis and his colleagues are to be commended for recognizing the overriding importance of culture in guiding the course of affectionate and respectful exchanges of behavior in personal relationships. Although some role theorists (e.g., McCall & Simmons, 1991) have acknowledged that ethnicity occupies a relatively high position in any hierarchy of behavioral influences, Triandis and colleagues have cast ethnicity in an even broader light. That is, for Triandis, ethnicity is tantamount to culture. In particular, Triandis has suggested that social scientists must consider familistic values in analyses of resource-giving (as well as resource-denying) behaviors among Latinas and Latinos. Using Triandis's concepts and results as a starting point, subsequent researchers may devise increasingly relationship-specific paradigms that document the patterns of *simpatia* and familism evident in Triandis's work.

One additional contribution by Triandis and his colleagues regarding social scientists' understanding of familism and the myth of machismo is more indirect yet worthy of comment. According to Gelfand, Triandis, and Chan (1996), collectivism—and, by extension within Triandis's framework, familism—generally has been conceptualized as the polar opposite of individualism. Furthermore, authoritarianism—which includes the pattern of male dominance popularly attributed to a "cult of masculinity" within Latina/o cultures—has been assumed to covary positively with collectivism and familism. However, Gelfand, Triandis, and Chan

(1996) reported that authoritarianism, like individualism, actually is unrelated to collectivism and familism. Instead, authoritarianism appears to represent the inverse of individualism. If authoritarianism is disentangled from concepts such as collectivism and familism, our contention that machismo can be distinguished from familism seems quite plausible.

Summary and Conclusions

To sum it up, we believe that the study of familism will yield unique insights into Latina/o personal relationships—insights that might not be obvious from a broadly collectivist framework, and insights that might not be obvious from prior research on non-Latino ethnic groups (Gaines, 1995b). Far from contradicting the results of Triandis and colleagues, however, it is precisely this clarity in conceptualization that may aid researchers in understanding why *simpatia* is so important as a Latina/o cultural value. Triandis's studies offer a promising glimpse into the future of research on familism and interpersonal resource exchange among Latinas and Latinos.

As we bring this chapter on Latina/Latino personal relationships to a close, we would be remiss if we did not consider the impact that Latinas/os' relatively young age at both marriage and parenthood is likely to have upon the personality and social development of all immediate family members through the years. Among Anglo families, the years beginning with the first child's entry into adolescence and ending with the last child's passage to adulthood are the years in which marital satisfaction is lowest. Not only do offspring undergo pronounced changes in self-evaluation, but parents change personally as well (Kimmel, 1974). Because Latinas/os tend to have their first children at an earlier age than do Anglos, the "turbulent years" may begin earlier in Latinas/os' family lives than in Anglos' family lives. Furthermore, because Latinas/os tend to have more children than do Anglo families, the "turbulent years" may last longer in Latino families than in Anglo families.

All of this seemingly would indicate that marital satisfaction tends to be lower among Latinas/os than among Anglos. However, Latina/o spouses are just as satisfied, on average, as are Anglo spouses (see Chilman, 1993; Suarez, 1993). How, if at all, does familism serve to buffer Latinas and Latinos from the inevitable stresses associated with family members' psychosocial development? Indeed, do Latina/o families undergo the same types of change as do Anglo families? Clinicians and researchers might find it profitable to explore the impact of prolonged generational conflicts on marital happiness, specifically within the context of affectionate and respectful behavior. Conversely, the benefits that multigenerational family interactions offer individuals might outweigh by far any potential costs accrued through marital and family interaction among Latinas and Latinos.

Finally, as Kimmel (1974) observed, ". . . family members have concepts of their *family* just as they have concepts of their *self*, and that the family concept may be measured in the same way that the self concept has been measured" (p. 197). Such an observation seems almost radical by conventional psychologists' standards, yet it is precisely this approach that holds the most promise for placing Latina/Latino personal relationships and interpersonal resource exchange in their proper context. Otherwise, basic and applied practitioners in the field of personal relationships may conclude—incorrectly—that Latina/o relationships are so "deviant" that they simply cannot be understood.

Preparation of this chapter was made possible by a postdoctoral fellowship from Franklin and Marshall College (1991–92), by a postdoctoral fellowship from the University of North Carolina at Chapel Hill (1992–93), by a postdoctoral fellowship from the Ford Foundation (1996–97), and by institutional funds from Pomona College from Pomona College to the first author. The authors are indebted to Hector Avalos, Steve Duck, Philip Rappaport, and two anonymous reviewers for their comments on an earlier version of this chapter.

4

Spiritualism and Personal Relationship Processes Among Asian American Couples

Despite the commonly held view that Asian Americans are a model minority who seemingly have achieved the "melting pot" ideal and the American dream, Asian Americans share with African Americans and Latinas/os the experience of prejudice and discrimination due to their unique heritage—and the experience of keeping alive a strong sense of cultural identity in the process (Hur & Proudlove, 1982). Few social scientists seem to be aware of the impact of discriminatory treatment (e.g., enactment of legislation such as the Chinese Exclusion Act and the Asian Exclusion Act; internment of Japanese Americans during World War II) upon the social and emotional lives upon Asian Americans (Bradshaw, 1994; Ou & McAdoo, 1993). In addition, many academicians in the United States have yet to acknowledge the array of obstacles still preventing many Asian Americans (e.g., Vietnamese refugees, Chinese sweatshop workers) from having the American Dream come true (Bradshaw, 1994; Tien, 1994).

What key values make Asian American culture distinctive? According to Cook and Kono (1977), one characteristic value is *spiritualism*, or an emphasis on understanding one's place within the natural order of the universe. This view is illustrated by the following: "The religious function of man becomes, not to alter . . . reality, but to learn to understand and accept it in the Hindu scheme, to comprehend one's present incarnation and prepare for a better one in the future, and in the Buddhist scheme, to become enlightened to the 'suchness' of existence" (Cook & Kono, 1977, p. 31). In this chapter, we shall consider this spiritualistic value orientation, as evident in Asian American patterns of interpersonal resource exchange in personal relationships.

Spiritualism Among Asian Americans

Ostensibly, individuals living in the United States whose ancestry can be traced to lands as diverse as China and the Philippines, Japan and India, and Korea and Vietnam all can be grouped together under the catchall term "Asian Americans." In reality, Asian Americans represent a variety of nations of origin, native languages, and religions (Bradshaw, 1994; Espiritu, 1992). Despite the fact that Asian Americans are a highly heterogeneous group, however, some authors (e.g., Min, 1995a; Wei, 1993) have argued that it is possible to identify certain cultural values that are shared by a plurality (if not an outright majority) of Americans with Asian ancestry. For the purposes of this chapter, we are interested especially in Eastern spiritualism, defined by Gilgen and Cho (1979) as follows:

> In summary, the Eastern perspective . . . is based on a non-dualistic view of reality which generates the following specific beliefs: (a) [M]an and nature are one; (b) the spiritual and physical are one; (c) mind and body are one; (d) man should recognize his basic oneness with nature, the spiritual, and the mental rather than attempt to analyze, categorize, manipulate, control, or consume the things of the world; (e) because of his oneness with all existence, man should feel "at home" in any place and with any person; (f) science and technology, at best, create an illusion of progress; (g) enlightenment involves achieving a sense of oneness with the universal; it is a state where all dichotomies vanish; and (h) meditation, a special state of quiet contemplation, is essential for achieving enlightenment. (p. 836)

According to Gilgen and Cho (1979), all four major Eastern religions (i.e., Hinduism, Buddhism, Confucianism, and

Taoism) emphasize the belief that humans cannot be separated conveniently into heavenly and earthly components (see also Braithwaite & Scott, 1991). Rather, heaven and earth form an indissoluble unity of which *Homo sapiens* is but one part. Furthermore, according to neo-Confucianist philosophy, human relationships involving significant others such as spouses, offspring, and friends are indispensable for maintaining order in the universe (see Chin, 1994). Interestingly, certain tenets of Eastern spiritualism (e.g., the self/other dichotomy is inherently false) have been embraced by scholars within the modern-day field of personal relationships (e.g., Aron & Aron, 1986, 1996).

This is not to say that the various Eastern religions differ in name only. For example, according to Bradshaw (1994), Buddhism addresses spiritual matters first and foremost, whereas Confucianism primarily addresses stability in social structure. Nevertheless, the four major Eastern religions all have common origins (Aron & Aron, 1986; Carter, 1995), which helps explain the relative ease with which elements of the seemingly disparate Eastern religions have been combined by some practitioners and philosophers (e.g., Wang Yang-ming's neo-Confucianism included elements of Buddhism, Taoism, and Confucianism; Miyuki, 1985a, b).

Cook and Kono (1977) suggested that spiritualism was as characteristic of Asian cultures as was individualism of European cultures and collectivism of African cultures (see also Myers, 1985). This does not mean that persons of European or African heritage inherently are less spiritualistic than are persons of Asian heritage (Jackson, 1983; Myers, 1985). At this point, I simply note that spiritualism is one cultural value orientation that might be useful in understanding interpersonal resource exchange and other personal relationship processes among Asian Americans.

Among the leading psychologists of the twentieth century, Carl Jung (e.g., Jung, 1978) was one of the few to acknowledge the importance of spiritualism (particularly the cluster of Eastern forms of spiritualism) as a potentially positive influence on individuals' personal and interpersonal well-being (Ewen, 1993; McClelland, 1987). Although Jung might be taken to task for "dipping into Eastern literature" (Aron & Aron, 1986, p. 6), Jung's analysis of spiritualism within the context of male-female relationships includes subtle nuances that probably would be lost upon more casual readers of Eastern philosophy.

In a neo-Confucian cosmology, the dialectics of *yin* and *yang* are manifested in multiple constructs (e.g., right-left, stillness-motion, male-female; see Miyuki, 1985a, b). From this neo-Confucianist cosmology, we might infer that the emotional and sexual intimacy arising between a man and a woman are the natural consequences of psychic unity or one-ness with the universe. In turn, the emotional and sexual intimacy arising between a man and a woman result in offspring, which serve to further strengthen the psychological bonds between the man and the woman.

Now let us examine Jung's explication of Eastern spiritualism in greater detail. Ironically, Jung consciously drew upon Hinduism, Buddhism, and Taoism but deliberately dismissed Confucianism—and, presumably, neo-Confucianism—as needlessly preoccupied with moral and social hierarchies (Clarke, 1992). Nevertheless, Jung's (1978) rendering of the concepts of *yin* and *yang* is quite compatible with that of neo-Confucianism philosophy:

> Spirit is something higher than intellect since it embraces the latter and includes the feelings as well. It is a guiding principle of life that strives towards superhuman, shining heights. Opposed to this *yang* principle is the dark, feminine, earthbound *yin*, whose emotionality and instinctuality reach back into the depths of time and down into the labyrinth of the physiological continuum. No doubt these are purely intuitive ideas, but one can hardly dispense with them if one is trying to understand the nature of the human psyche. The Chinese could not do without them because, as the history of Chinese philosophy shows, they never strayed so far from the central psychic facts as to lose themselves in a one-sided over-development and over-valuation of a single function. They never failed to acknowledge the paradoxicality and polarity of all life. The opposites always balanced one another—a sign of high culture. One-sidedness, though it lends momentum, is a mark of barbarism. (p. 11)

Jung's interpretation of *yin* and *yang* suggests that femininity and masculinity in and of themselves are not inherently good. Instead, whether at the level of the individual or of the entire culture, human beings should strive to incorporate femininity *and* masculinity into their social-psychological lives. Consistent with Jung, theorists and researchers in social/personality psychology (e.g., Spence, Helmreich, & Holahan, 1979; see also Gaines, 1995a; Wiggins, 1991) increasingly have noted that excessive reliance on femininity or masculinity—particularly in their socially undesirable or negative forms—can have deleterious consequences for cultures and personalities alike.

Perhaps the most important Jungian concepts for our purposes are those of *animus* (i.e., the element of masculinity found in women) and *anima* (i.e., the element of femininity found in men; Ewen, 1993). Jung believed that although male-female attraction certainly involves a large sexual component (de Beauvoir, 1953), much of the basis for attraction between men and women involves a large spiritual component as well. According to Jung, men and women possess the capacity to understand each other at a deep spiritual level because both men and women are masculine *and* feminine by nature (Ewen, 1993). In fact, the reason that miscommunication commonly occurs between men and women (Tannen, 1990; see also Gaines, 1994a; Ickes, 1993) is not so much because the two sexes have been socialized so differently, but rather because socialization often prevents men from unearthing their *anima* and women from unearthing their *animus* from beneath layers of unconsciousness.

Extending Jung's analysis of *animus* and *anima* to the study of interpersonal resource exchange, we might conclude that women and men will reciprocate affection to the extent that (a) men acknowledge that they need affection (a stereotypically "feminine" commodity) as well as respect; (b) women acknowledge that they need respect (a stereotypically "masculine" commodity) as well as affection; (c) men respond to women's need for both affection and respect; and (d) women respond to men's need for both affection and respect. Jung's (1978) spiritualistic analysis also implies that sexual intimacy does not presuppose socioemotional intimacy and vice versa, a point made by resource exchange theorists (e.g., L'Abate & Harel, 1991) and by scholars of Eastern spiritualism (e.g., Lebra, 1994). Although critics of Jung frequently have viewed spiritualism as antithetical to psychological well-being (if not antithetical to psychology as a science; see Moacanin, 1986), Jung's perspective—buttressed by research on the psychometric properties of measures of spiritualism (e.g., Gilgen & Cho, 1979; see also Braithwaite & Scott, 1991)—lends legitimacy to the study of spiritualism as a potential predictor of patterns of emotional intimacy among Asian Americans.

Implicit in our examination of spiritualism is the assumption that Eastern religions constitute an important part of culture and ethnic identity for many persons of Asian descent in the United States (see Carter, 1995; Tamura, 1994). Of course, it would be inaccurate to suggest that all Asian Americans embrace Eastern spiritualism, particularly when one considers the significance of Christianity among persons of Korean descent (Kitano & Daniels, 1988). Nevertheless, it is possible that Eastern spiritualism permeates the relational lives of Asian Americans to a greater extent than is the case for Anglos (or, for that matter, African Americans and Latinas/os).

One intriguing statistic that is consistent with such a contention is the relatively low divorce rates of Asian American couples, compared with the divorce rates of all other major ethnic groups. Some authors (e.g., del Carmen, 1990) have concluded that the low divorce rate is a consequence of Asian American couples' adherence to traditional Confucian norms of male privilege (e.g., in Confucian societies, women could not obtain a divorce, no matter how badly they were mistreated by their husbands). However, perhaps the low divorce rate largely reflects high levels of spiritualism. Unfortunately, studies of Asian American marriage and divorce patterns tend to concentrate on demographics (e.g., proportion of Asian Americans who marry persons who are/are not of Asian ancestry), rather than partners' motives for staying married or getting divorced.

Unlike the stereotypes that are evoked commonly in American society's depictions of African Americans (see Chapter 2) and of Latinas/os (Chapter 3), the stereotypes of Asian American couples frequently suggest that neither men nor women influence each other's behavior to a large degree. It is almost as if Asian American relationships *per se* do not even exist in the eyes of American society. In the following two sections, I shall examine the stereotypes regarding Asian American men as passive and Asian American women as exotic.

Stereotypes: Passive Men

Of all the stereotypes applied wantonly to men of various ethnic groups, perhaps the least flattering are those applied to Asian American men. Hollywood has offered two enduring stereotypic images of Asian American men: The hypersexual Fu Manchu and the asexual Charlie Chan (Marchetti, 1993; Wei, 1993; Wilson & Gutierrez, 1985). At a surface level, the two stereotypes appear to be polar opposites, despite Chan's apparent heterosexuality—how else are we to account for Chan's "Number One Son"? At a deeper level, however, neither Fu Manchu nor Charlie Chan emerges as a potent sex symbol. Rather, both are caricatures devoid of sex appeal (Espiritu, 1997; see also Okihiro, 1994).

In everyday life, Asian American men seem to be held up to the passive Charlie Chan stereotype far more often than to the hyperaggressive Fu Manchu stereotype (Lee, 1991; O'Brien & Fugita, 1991). In fact, the model minority stereotype—that of Asian Americans as obsessed with educational and financial success—often evokes images of Asian American men as computer nerds whose intellectual prowess overshadows their physical prowess. As Wei (1993) observed, Charlie Chan is the epitome of the model minority stereotype:

> [Charlie] Chan, supposed to be a well-educated immigrant with a mastery of both Eastern and Western knowledge, had the quaint habit of speaking English as if he had learned it from reading aphorisms found in fortune cookies. Yet he was supposed to be a positive portrayal! That is, he represented a European American's ideal image of an Asian American projected on the silver screen: Intelligent, passive, polite, self-effacing, and effeminate. With the possible exception of intelligence, none of his vaunted attributes ranked high on the American scale of manhood. Small wonder that Asian American cultural nationalists, particularly men, were offended. Equally galling was the fact that in forty-seven feature-length movies, Charlie Chan had been played by European American actors; though his sons were played by Asian Americans. (p. 52)

Indirect evidence with regard to the influence of such stereotypes on women's perceptions of Asian American men as potential dating or marriage partners comes from a variety of sources. For example, Tucker and Mitchell-Kernan (1995) reported that Asian American men were more likely to be excluded by African American women and Latinas than were men of any other ethnic group (among the 26% of African American women who would exclude certain men from consideration, 52% explicitly excluded Asian American men; among the 41% of Latinas who would exclude certain men from consideration, 44% explicitly excluded Asian American men). Furthermore, even though 70% of all Asian Americans in California marry within the same racial (and, usually, the same national) group (Shinagawa & Pang, 1988), Asian American women are three times more likely to marry outside their racial group than are Asian American men in California (Kitano, Yeung, Chai, & Hatanaka, 1984). Some social scientists view the latter statistic as evidence that even some Asian American women explicitly reject Asian American men in response to prevailing stereotypes regarding Asian American men as passive (e.g., Espiritu, 1997; Serafica, 1990).

Whether the above statistics regarding the desirability of Asian American men as potential romantic partners actually reflect women's internalized stereotypes of Asian American men is subject to debate. For example, Agbayani-Siewert and Revilla (1995) noted that some social scientists have attributed Asian American men's presumed lack of desirability to Asian American men's sexism; Min (1995b) countered that many traditional Asian American men might actively avoid relationships with nontraditional women. Nevertheless, subjective accounts from some Asian American men (see Lee, 1991; O'Brien & Fugita, 1992) indicate that they have been stigmatized by the Charlie Chan-like, asexual images that have pervaded twentieth-century American media (Guerrero, 1993; Marchetti, 1993; Wei, 1993; Wilson & Gutierrez, 1985). Thus, within the realm of personal relationships, the "model minority" stereotype has been none too flattering to Asian American men.

What need, if any, does the Charlie Chan stereotype fulfill within the American psyche? One possibility is that such a stereotype obscures historical instances of discrimination, such as legislation in the United States that effectively denied the access of Asian American men to wives of *any* ethnicity for many years. Fisher (1980) described some of these discriminatory efforts:

The first Asians to immigrate to the United States were the Chinese. In the wake of a severe drought that destroyed the crops in the Canton province in 1847 to 1850, many Chinese came over to work on the Central Railroad, trying to earn enough money to return to China, and in light of the enormous expense of the trip, most men did not bring wives or families with them. The results were long, arduous separations that often threatened the family unit and made life painfully difficult on both sides of the Pacific. Women were left behind in small villages with barely enough resources to survive and the responsibility of caring for their families alone. Those few who were able to break tradition encountered an even bleaker life of poverty and hard work in the United States. In many instances, single women venturing the long voyage alone to join their husbands were kidnapped and sold into prostitution. The Chinese Exclusion Act of 1882, which prohibited immigration by laborers, increased the difficulties for women because, as wives of laborers, they were denied entry to the United States. By 1890 Chinese women in the United States numbered only 3,869 in comparison to 103,620 men. It was not until 1943 that the Exclusion Act was repealed and many Chinese wives and their children were permitted to enter the United States. Reversing its previous policy and now intent on "promoting family unity," the government also passed the Amended War Brides Act in 1947, which allowed more Chinese wives to immigrate. . . .

In short, Americas streets were not golden, and opportunities were meager in a country that continued to discriminate against [Asian Americans]: In 1913 the Alien Land Law Act was passed, which prevented Asians from owning land in California, and in 1924 the Asian Exclusion Act, which prohibited intermarriage between Asians and whites and denied citizenship rights to Chinese and Japanese, became law. (pp. 433–435)

It was not until 1948 that the California Supreme Court struck down the Asian Exclusion Act as unconstitutional (Lee, 1991); and even the original War Brides Act of 1945 primarily benefited European and, eventually, Asian wives of White U.S. servicemen (Thornton, 1992). Overall, large numbers of Asian American men effectively were barred from intraethnic as well as interethnic marriages long before the image of Charlie Chan became a fixture in American popular culture (Lyman, 1994). Such facts belie the notion that Asian American men somehow have been inept at forming and sustaining romantic heterosexual relationships.

Amazingly, some social scientists (e.g., Webster, 1992) have disputed the conclusion that American legislative decisions directly affecting Asian American men and women were racist. Given the preponderance of evidence regarding White American fears of a "yellow peril" throughout the first half of the twentieth century (Lee, 1991), it is difficult to deny either the intent or the effects of the Chinese Exclusion Act or the Asian Exclusion Act regarding the ability of Asian American men historically to marry and raise families in the United States. Only by denying the pervasive and continuing importance of race in American society is it possible to minimize the racist implications of such explicitly anti-Asian American legislation (see Lyman, 1994; Wilson & Gutierrez, 1985).

Stereotypes: Exotic Women

In stark contrast to the stereotyped image of Asian American men as sexless, Hollywood frequently portrays Asian American women as exotic sex objects who will do anything to please their men (Marchetti, 1993; Wei, 1993; Wilson & Gutierrez, 1985). Interestingly, in numerous American films and television series, Asian American women are more likely to be stereotyped as the "property" of White men than of Asian American men. In many such Hollywood creations, Asian American men are totally absent.

Perhaps the most enduring stereotype of the Asian/Asian American woman as sex goddess is that of Suzie Wong. The fictitious Suzie (played in the movie by Nancy Kwan) is a "fallen woman" (i.e., prostitute) living in Hong Kong who ultimately falls in love with a White male artist, Robert Lomax (played by William Holden), from the United States. In *The World of Suzie Wong*, the "White man's burden" of saving Suzie from a life of moral and romantic despair is played to maximum effect. As Marchetti (1993) pointed out, Suzie

Wong's world is a not-so-subtle metaphor for the Third World as a whole:

[In *The World of Suzie Wong,*] Hong Kong provides a place where all sorts of social and ideological oppositions can be played out in fiction—East-West, Communist-capitalist, white-nonwhite, rich-poor, colonizer-colonized, European-American, Asian-American, progressive-conservative. Within the context of the Hollywood love story, moreover, all these oppositions can be addressed using the cinematic vocabulary of that fundamental opposition between male and female. By using the romance to examine these other ideological sore points, Hollywood can make any boundaries between nations and races appear as natural as the differences between men and women. Relationships between nations or races can be seen as the male-female relationship writ large, with its patronizing sentimentality and inherent inequality left intact. (p. 110)

Suzie's salvation in *The World of Suzie Wong* is . . . literal, clearly affirming Western liberalism's claim to be able to criticize itself and press on for the good of "humanity." In the climactic scene in which a flood causes a landslide in the slum where Suzie's baby lives, Suzie seeks out Robert's help. Both struggle in vain to save the baby, and, through this lost battle, Robert, in fact, manages to save Suzie from the last emotional link she had with the slums of Hong Kong. At the baby's funeral, Robert and Suzie reaffirm their love, and she is effectively "saved" from returning to the world of prostitution, which led to this initial, tragic, failed domesticity. She is "free" to begin again under the protection of her white knight. Robert has a moral right to fulfill this role. As the "enlightened" American artist, he is positioned above the hypocrisy of the British (i.e., the sailors and Ben, who either brutalize or exploit Suzie) and the cruelty of the Asian male (the baby's unseen, but villainous father). Patriarchal, white, and American moral prerogatives, therefore, all neatly come together as the couple walk off into the distance at the film's end. (pp. 116–117)

Just as Fu Manchu looms as a counterpoint to the Charlie Chan stereotype applied to Asian American men, so too does a thoroughly evil stereotype—that of the Dragon Lady—sometimes emerge as a counterpoint to the ostensibly benign yet ultimately harmful Suzie Wong stereotype applied to Asian American women (Bradshaw, 1994). With the relatively recent ascendancy of the Asian American feminist movement, it is possible that the Dragon Lady stereotype will be invoked increasingly in American popular culture in the years to come. Nevertheless, the Suzie Wong stereotype is likely to retain considerable popularity in American society, precisely because it is so reassuring in the minds of many Anglos (Bradshaw, 1994; Espiritu, 1997; Marchetti, 1993).

Just how pervasive is the Suzie Wong stereotype? One need look no further than commercial advertisements to find Suzie Wong alive and well, even in the post-Civil Rights era. In a study of representations of persons of color in American mass media, Wilson and Gutierrez (1985) listed several instances in which women of Asian descent were depicted as exotic yet accessible:

> Companies pitching everything from pantyhose to airlines featured Asian women coiffed and consumed as seductive China dolls to promote their products, some of them draped in a Chinese setting and others attentively caring for the needs of the Anglo men in the advertisement. One airline boasted that those who flew with it would be under the care of the "Singapore girl."
>
> Asian women appearing in commercials are often featured as China dolls, with the small, darkened eyes, straight hair with bangs, and a narrow slit skirt. Another common portrayal features the exotic, tropical Pacific Islands look, complete with flowers in the hair, a sarong or grass skirt, and shell ornamentation. Asian women hoping to become models have sometimes found that they must conform to these stereotypes or lose assignments. One Asian American model was told to cut her hair with bangs when she auditioned for a beer advertisement. When she refused, the beer company decided to hire another model with shorter hair cut in bangs. (pp. 118–119)

As Madison Avenue often proclaims, "Sex sells"—and what better embodiment of female sexuality to exploit than

Suzie Wong? Conspicuously absent in the aforementioned advertisements are husbands or boyfriends, especially those of Asian ancestry. Instead, Asian American women typically are presented as sexy, single, and available to Anglo men only.

Theoretical Perspectives on
Asian American Relationships

Given the preponderance of stereotypes regarding Asian American men as passive and of Asian American women as exotic, what predictions might be made using a stereotyped model of interpersonal resource exchange among Asian American couples? Furthermore, how might such a model differ from a spiritualistic model, in which Eastern spiritualism is hypothesized to be manifested in exchanges of affectionate and/or respectful behavior among Asian American couples? In this section, I consider the competing claims of stereotyped and spiritualistic models of interpersonal resource exchange among Asian American heterosexual couples.

Using a stereotyped frame of reference in trying to predict patterns of interpersonal resource exchange among Asian American couples, we might expect that Asian American men and women seldom display affection or respect to each other in the first place. Thus, Asian American men and women would not have the opportunity to influence each other; their interpersonal worlds would be too separate to allow much meaningful dialogue to take place. The stereotyped model of interpersonal resource exchange among Asian Americans is shown in Figure 4.1.

In contrast, using a spiritualistic frame of reference, we might expect that Asian American men and women in ongoing relationships tend to reciprocate affection and respect to the extent that individuals' attitudes and beliefs reflect precepts of Eastern spiritualism. In making this prediction, we draw upon Aron and Aron's (1986) conceptualization of love as an expansion of self, as well as Wiggins's (1991) conceptualization of agency and communion as part of a (neo-)Confucian world view. The spiritualistic model of interpersonal resource exchange among Asian American couples is presented in Figure 4.2.

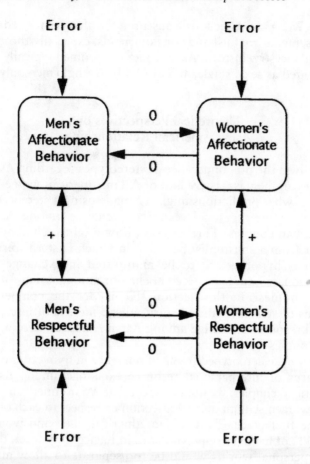

Figure 4.1:
Stereotyped model of interpersonal resource exchange among Asian American couples

At first glance, the spiritualistic model described above might seem antithetical to the actual practice of Eastern religions in Asia and in America. For example, some authors (e.g., del Carmen, 1990; Gold, 1993; Kibria, 1993; Matsui, 1989) have associated Confucianism, Hinduism, Buddhism, and Taoism with male privilege and asymmetrical marital relationships. However, other authors (e.g., Bradshaw, 1994; see also C. Lin & W. T. Liu, 1993; Taylor & Arbuckle, 1995; Yu & Yang, 1994) have countered by suggesting that the *in-*

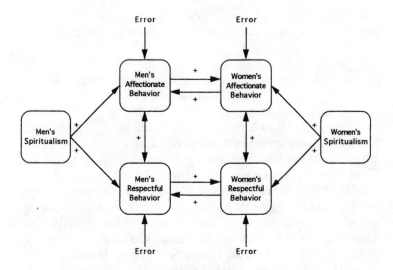

Figure 4.2:
*Spiritualistic model of interpersonal resource exchange
among Asian American couples*

stitutionalization of Eastern religions—most notably Confucianism—codified male privilege far more rigidly than the basic philosophies underlying those religions would suggest.

Interestingly, Lebra (1994) concluded that it was only *after* ridding itself of Confucian political doctrine in the years
following World War II (see Iwao, 1993) that Japan became a
truly spiritual nation. Moreover, Bradshaw (1994) concluded
that *Western* imperialism was as detrimental to women's status in Asian nations as was Eastern imperialism. Also, it is
clear that Eastern beliefs about spirituality *per se* (e.g., "I do
not believe in a personal god"; "If there is a soul, I believe that
after I die it will lose its individuality and become one with the
overall spirituality of the universe") are not synonymous with
beliefs about male superiority (Gilgen & Cho, 1979).

The study by Gelfand, Triandis, and Chan (1996) mentioned in Chapters 1 and 3 of this volume offers indirect support for the view that spiritualism is distinct from
androcentrism. Gelfand et al. found that "devoutness"—
which they described as one component of collectivism, but
which I would term *spiritualism*—was unrelated to author-

itarianism. In turn, I would describe the notion of male superiority as a major component of authoritarianism.

Empirical Research on Asian American Relationships

Although Asian Americans constitute the United States's fastest-growing group of persons of color, empirical research on personal relationships among Asian Americans hardly reflects that population growth (Gaines, 1995b; Staples & Mirande, 1980). Actual studies of Asian American relationships are few and far between. Most studies of relationships among persons of Asian ancestry have been conducted outside the United States (e.g., Durrett, Richards, Otaki, Pennebaker, & Nyquist, 1986; Edwards, Fuller, Sermsri, & Vorakitphokatorn, 1992; Goldman, 1993; Rindfuss, Liao, & Tsuya, 1992; Roopnairne, Talukder, Jain, Joshi, & Srivastav, 1992; Shukla, 1987; Stack, 1992; Xiaohe & Whyte, 1990). Even those that examine Asian Americans typically compare demographic trends, such as intraracial and interracial marriage rates (e.g., Johnson & Nagoshi, 1986; Kitano, Yeung et al., 1984; Labov & Jacobs, 1986; Schoen & Thomas, 1989; Shinagawa & Pang, 1988) rather than partners' thoughts, feelings, or behavior. Is it possible, then, to find *any* empirical studies that focus on personal relationship processes among Asian Americans? If so, how relevant are those studies regarding spiritualism and interpersonal resource exchange among Asian Americans?

In a qualitative study of marital relationships in Japan, Iwao (1993) argued that of all personal relationships, the husband-wife relationship is most likely to involve reciprocation of affectionate and respectful behaviors—at least within the home—because it is the least scripted of all relationships. Iwao attributed the relative success of Japanese marriages in part to Confucian and Buddhist teachings regarding human beings as imperfect, constantly expanding, and in continual need of bolstering self-love and self-respect via the affection and respect given by spouses. Iwao's (1993) analysis, then, is consistent with the spiritualistic model of interpersonal resource exchange between partners of Asian ancestry living in the United States.

In a review of the literature on relationships among Filipino Americans, Agbayani-Siewert and Revilla (1995) cited spiritualism as a positive influence on male-female relationships (see also Bradshaw, 1994). Interestingly, Confucianism and Hinduism are not typically embraced by Filipino Americans to the same extent as by other Asian American groups (for further discussions of the sociocultural and sociohistorical differences among persons of Filipino ancestry and persons of other Asian ancestry, see Espiritu, 1992; Kitano & Daniels, 1988). Nevertheless, the type of spiritualism embraced by many Filipino Americans is *not* Jewish or Christian; the form of spiritualism described by Agbayani-Siewert and Revilla (1995) is decidedly Eastern in its origins:

> The Filipino family is structured differently from other Asian groups in the distribution of authority and power. . . . Unlike other Asian groups, family authority [among Filipino Americans] is not patriarchal, but more egalitarian, where husband and wife share almost equally in financial and family decisions. . . . Unlike Judeo-Christian explanations of Eve being created from the rib of Adam, a Filipino legend has both man and woman emerging simultaneously from a large bamboo tube. . . . Filipino descendants are traced bilaterally through both parents. (p. 160)

By the same token, not all studies on Asian Americans offer such a favorable impression of the link between spiritualism and personal relationship processes. For instance, some studies of domestic violence among Vietnamese American couples (e.g., Kibria, 1993) have implicated Confucianism as a *negative* influence on affectionate and respectful behaviors. That is, the male-dominated hierarchy advocated by Confucius (see Bradshaw, 1994; Cha, 1994) encouraged female dependency upon men from birth until death (upon fathers, then upon husbands, and then upon sons).

Among those Vietnamese American couples who continue to follow Confucian doctrine, such dependency may encourage women to lavish affection and respect upon men but not vice versa. Not all scholars of Vietnamese Americans would blame Confucianism in and of itself, however. For example, Kitano and Daniels (1988) commented that among traditional Vietnamese American families, individuals frequently complain about "the high value placed on work and achievement over interpersonal relationships" (p. 143) *in American society.*

Research on Korean American relationships illustrates the difficulties that can arise in attempting to attribute patterns of socioemotional intimacy (or lack thereof) to Eastern spiritualism. According to Min (1995b), for instance, Confucianism dictates strict hierarchical relations between Korean American husbands and wives (i.e., women's giving of respect toward men but not vice versa), apparently with no provision for affectionate behavior on the part of either gender. However, Cha (1994) argued that "If hierarchy stands for the vertical dimension of in-group relationships, dependence and *chong* [i.e., affection] are the glue that binds individual members together in traditional Korea" (p. 166).

Cha distinguished between those Korean cultural values that emphasize mutuality in affection and respect (e.g., *chong, ch'inbun,* and *uichi*) and those Korean values that emphasize asymmetry in power relations (e.g., *ye, bunsu,* and *ch'ung-hyo*). Min (1993) conceived of spiritualism among Korean American couples as primarily Confucian and as *discouraging* exchanges of affection and respect, whereas Cha (1994) conceived of spiritualism among those couples as primarily Confucian but as *encouraging* exchanges involving affection and respect, at least to some degree. Complicating matters even further, Kitano and Daniels (1988) contended that Christianity in general (and Catholicism in particular) had supplanted Confucianism as the primary form of spiritualism among Korean Americans, thus raising the question as to whether Confucianism is reflected at all in patterns of interpersonal resource exchange among Korean American couples.

Aside from the issue of whether Confucianism is significantly and/or negatively related to reciprocity of affection and respect among Korean American couples, Min (1993, 1995b) called attention to the need for researchers to determine whether particular pairings involve (a) Korean-born men with Korean-born women, (b) Korean-born men with U.S.-born women, (c) U.S.-born men with Korean-born women, or (d) U.S.-born men with U.S.-born women. Min speculated that conflict would be greater among couples in which spouses came from different countries than among couples in which spouses came from the same country. In particular, marriages involving partners from different countries presumably were especially likely to have been arranged (and, therefore, less likely to have been formed as the result of mutual love or affection). Moreover, Min suggested that conflict would be greater among couples involving Korean-born men with U.S.-born women than among couples involving U.S.-born men with Korean-born women. In particular, Korean-born men presumably were especially likely to have married U.S.-born women specifically to emigrate to the United States (subsequently divorcing those women so that they, in turn, could become U.S. citizens, return to Korea long enough to marry their "true" loves, and then emigrate to the United States to stay).

Thus far, Min's (1993, 1995b) predictions have not been verified empirically. Nevertheless, Min's point concerning the cross-national aspect of many Asian American marriages is important. For example, marriages between Chinese and Japanese immigrants, or between first-generation Vietnamese Americans and second-generation Korean Americans, conceivably could reflect the influence of multiple forms of Eastern spiritualism upon patterns of interpersonal resource exchange.

In considering empirical studies of spiritualism and interpersonal resource exchange among Asian American couples, it is important not to overlook the socioeconomic and sociohistorical forces that have affected the availability of same-race (if not same-ethnicity) mates for Asian American men in particular. At various times during the nineteenth and twentieth centuries, large numbers of Chinese, Japanese, Korean, Vietnamese, Filipino, and other men from Asia moved to the United States in hopes of finding economic independence. Many of those men were married and were forced to leave their wives and children behind for many years—or forever. Furthermore, those Asian men who emigrated to the United States without having been married first in their native countries not only found few available Asian American women but also were prevented legally from marrying Anglo women. To the extent that male chauvinism emerged in the "bachelor communities" that subsequently developed, then, one might wonder whether chauvinism occurred *despite* or *because of* their sojourn to America (see Lyman, 1994; Okihiro, 1994).

Returning to contemporary empirical studies relevant to spiritualism and reciprocity of affection and respect among Asian American couples, relationship researchers are just beginning to develop and test theories regarding East-West cultural differences and associated interpersonal behaviors. Perhaps not surprisingly, relationship researchers have begun to amass a mixed bag of empirical results. For instance, let us take the concept of *agape*—selfless, spiritual love—which is described by Lee (1976) as one of six possible "love styles" (see also Aron & Aron, 1986; Duck, 1992; Fehr, 1993, 1994). On the one hand, Aron and Aron (1986) noted that although the concept can be found in all of the world's major religions, *agape* does not appear to be manifested strongly in personal relationships in Western nations. On the other hand, Sprecher et al. (1994) reported that *agape* was higher in a sample of predominantly European American women and men than in a sample of Japanese women and men.

It is not clear from the study by Sprecher et al. (1994) whether the links between *agape* and relational processes such as reciprocal liking were higher in the American sample or in the Japanese sample. Sprecher et al. conducted analyses of variance, using gender and nationality as predictors of personality characteristics and relational processes. However, they did not report the correlations between *agape* and reciprocal liking. Also, although Sprecher et al.'s (1994) American sample (*n* = 1043) included 94 Asian Americans, comparisons between Asians' and Asian Americans' scores on *agape* and reciprocal liking were not reported.

In a study of cultural and ethnic influences on personal relationship processes among various American ethnic groups, Doherty, Hatfield, Thompson, and Choo (1994) hypothesized that European Americans would be more individualistic than Japanese Americans, Pacific Islanders, or Chinese Americans. Following Dion and Dion (1993), Doherty et al. also hypothesized that European Americans would experience higher levels of both passionate and companionate love than would any of the Asian American ethnic groups. As it turned out, European Americans were more individualistic yet *lower* in self-reported passionate and companionate love than were any of the Asian American groups. Individualism also proved to be negatively correlated with passionate and companionate love, although the magnitude of the correlations was well below .20 in absolute value.

An important limitation of many studies on East-West differences in spiritualism and personal relationship processes is that key concepts within Eastern cultures have been ignored by many, if not most, American social psychologists (Doherty et al., 1994; Sprecher et al., 1994). For instance, Dion and Dion (1993) argued that the concept of *amae*, which reflects one's desire to "be a passive love object and to be indulged by another" (p. 56) and is central to Japanese culture, has no equivalent in Western nations. *Amae* captures both the self-in-relationship quality of interpersonal resource exchange and the self-in-the-universe quality of spiritualism, yet this concept has yet to be measured explicitly in empirical studies of personal relationship processes. Researchers' failure to measure *amae* and related concepts may hinder efforts at predicting relational dynamics among persons of Asian heritage (Lin & Rusbult, 1995).

Summary and Conclusions

In this chapter, I have commented on the promise that a spiritualistic model of interpersonal resource exchange holds for understanding relationship processes among Asian American couples. To date, no definitive study of spiritualism and reciprocity of affection and respect in Asian American male-female relationships has been conducted. In the remainder of this chapter, I offer a series of recommendations for enterprising researchers who wish to test the spiritualistic, stereotypic, and/or other models of interpersonal resource exchange and related processes among Asian American couples.

First, researchers should explicitly measure spiritualism, preferably in its Eastern forms (e.g., Confucianism/neo-Confucianism, Taoism, Buddhism, Hinduism). It is tempting to assume that persons of Asian heritage are uniformly high in spiritualism and low in individualism (see Kamo, 1993). However, it is possible that any link between degree of Asian ancestry and personal relationship processes will be mediated by spiritualism and related cultural value orientations (see Doherty et al., 1994). It is also possible that links between spiritualism and interpersonal resource exchange will be moderated by ethnicity, such that spiritualism as a significant positive predictor of individuals' displays of affectionate and respectful behaviors toward their partners is especially pronounced among Asian Americans (see Gaines, 1995b).

Second, researchers will have to make finer distinctions between spiritualism and other "we orientations" than have been made in previous studies. In most research comparing Anglos' and Asian Americans' cultural values, it is assumed that collectivism encompasses Asian Americans' orientations toward community, family, and a higher natural order (Dion & Dion, 1993). However, given the difficulty that many Asian Americans have experienced in attempting to forge a sense of unity among persons of Chinese, Japanese, Korean, Filipino, and Vietnamese descent (Espiritu, 1992), it may be inaccurate to depict collectivism in its more limited sense (i.e., as an orientation toward the welfare of one's larger community) as a distinctly Asian American value (Cook & Kono, 1977).

Unlike African Americans (most of whom are English monolingual and were born in the United States) or Latinas/os (most of whom are Spanish-English bilingual but who may have been born in the United States, Mexico, Puerto Rico, Cuba, or a number of Central or South American nations), the twenty or so nationalities lumped together under the term "Asian Americans" represent a variety of linguistic groups (Wilkinson, 1993). Also, given the restrictive U.S. immigration laws that left generations of Asian immigrant men without their wives and girlfriends from back home (Lyman, 1994; Okihiro, 1994), it may be inaccurate to depict an orientation toward the welfare of one's immediate and extended family as a distinctly Asian American value. In contrast, the belief in self-in-relation-to-the-universe unifies the otherwise disparate forms of Eastern spiritualism likely to be manifested in Asian Americans' relational behaviors (see Aron & Aron, 1986).

Third, researchers should be careful not to assume that spiritualism necessarily entails endorsement of male privilege in Asian American relationships. Throughout American history, women of every ethnicity have been accorded less status than have their male counterparts (Allman, 1996). The notion that Confucianism is uniquely indicative of power differentials favoring men, for example, belies the fact that even among Protestant White couples in the United States, finding marriages in which husbands and wives continue to follow traditional gender-role arrangements is relatively easy (Ickes, 1993; Johnson, Huston, Gaines, & Levinger, 1992). This is not to deny Confucius's own pronouncements regarding male superiority. I simply note that in and of itself, Eastern spiritualism is not inherently sexist (see Bradshaw, 1994).

Finally, I emphasize the need for researchers to consider spiritualism and personal relationship processes among Asian American couples *in their own right*, rather than inevitably compared with corresponding processes among Anglo couples. By refraining from casting judgment upon Asian American relationship processes as deviating from Anglo relational norms, researchers might discover that concepts such as *amae* are unique to Asian American couples (Dion & Dion, 1993; Y. W Lin & Rusbult, 1995). By the same token, perhaps researchers will find that some issues, such as those regarding fairness in interpersonal resource exchange, are not nearly as salient among Asian ancestry couples as they are among Anglo couples (Kamo, 1993). I hasten to add that judging Asian American relationship processes as "unique" requires at least a modicum of knowledge regarding counterparts (e.g., Anglo relationship processes). Nonetheless, perhaps researchers will begin to examine similarities and differences *within* this heterogeneous group, in addition to examining similarities and differences between Asian Americans and Anglos *per se*.

In this and preceding chapters, I have focused almost exclusively upon cultural value orientations and interpersonal resource exchange among heterosexual couples involving partners from the same racial/ethnic background. In the next chapter, however, we shall shift our focus to relationships involving interethnic/interracial couples. We have already alluded to relationships involving Anglos paired with Asian Americans. In Chapter 5, we will pay particular attention to the least frequent yet most controversial of all interethnic/interracial relationships—Black-White relationships, especially Black male-White female relationships. As we shall see, even when relationships involve partners who are not of the same ethnicity, certain cultural value orientations may help establish and maintain satisfying patterns of behavior.

Preparation of this chapter was facilitated by a postdoctoral fellowship from the Ford Foundation (1996–97), and by institutional funds from Pomona College. The author wishes to thank David Kwon and Nancy Yum for their help in obtaining articles to be reviewed for this chapter. The author also is indebted to Ruth Chung for her comments on earlier versions of this chapter.

5

Romanticism and Interpersonal Resource Exchange Among Interethnic Couples

Stanley O. Gaines, Jr., and James H. Liu

Prior to World War II, a sociopolitical movement captured the hearts and minds of many Europeans and European Americans—the eugenics movement. Triggered in large part by fears that "mongrel" races were breeding at an excessively large rate, this movement was given a quasi-scientific legitimacy by some sociologists, biologists, and psychologists of the day. In fact, no less a figure than Leonard Darwin (son of Charles Darwin) spelled out the goals of eugenics explicitly: "We can at all events assert that there are many kinds of men that we do not want. These include the criminal, the insane, the imbecile, the feeble in mind, the diseased at birth, the deformed, the deaf, the blind, etc., etc." (1929, p. 25). Belonging to the "etc., etc." category were the products of "miscegenation" or "race mixing," according to Osborn (1923): "In the matter of racial virtues, my opinion is that from biological principles there is little evidence in the 'melting pot' theory. Put three races together, you are as likely to unite the vices of all three as the virtues" (p. 2).

Although the eugenics movement eventually became distasteful to many social scientists and politicians as Nazism ran its course during the 1930s and 1940s (Howitt & Owusu-Bempah, 1994), followers of that movement touched

a nerve in the American psyche.[1] Few taboos have generated
as many myths, consternation, or outright violence as have the
taboos against sexual relations between persons classified socially as belonging to different "races," especially within the
context of marriage (Gaines & Ickes, 1997). It is remarkable
that, in a society where sex traditionally has been *reserved* for
marriage in theory if not in practice, many Anglo males in particular have been encouraged to avoid "getting serious" with
sexual partners *when those partners are of ethnicities different
from their own* (Sanjek, 1994; Washington, 1970).[2]

Nevertheless it is clear that, in full defiance of American
social mores (and, often, in defiance of the law; see Spickard,
1989), many men and women differing in ethnicity have con-
summated their relationships throughout the centuries. For
instance, as many as 75% of all persons classified as Black in
the United States have one of more ancestors classified as
White (Allport, 1954; Gordon, 1964; Porterfield, 1978; Root,
1992). In neighboring Mexico, as many as 80% of all persons
are products of "mesticization" (i.e., the physical and cultural
union of European and Native ancestry; see Porterfield, 1978;
Ramirez, 1983; Root, 1992). In Hawaii, the extent of race
mixing and cultural diversity historically has been so great
that some observers have referred to that state as "the show-
place of American democracy" (see Adams, 1937; but see
also Lyman, 1994).

If America's ethnic groups differ in relative emphasis on
a variety of cultural values (as has been argued throughout

---

[1]This is not to imply that the eugenics movement is extinct. As
Steve Duck (personal communication, 1992) informed us, "There is
still a large and active Eugenics Society in the U.K. I rejected an in-
vitation to speak there in 1983."

[2]In this chapter, we use the terms "interethnic" and "interracial" as if they were synonymous. Some authors (e.g., Crohn, 1995)
have argued that racial groups do not constitute ethnic groups *per
se*; other authors (e.g., Gaines, 1995b) have maintained that race is
part and parcel of ethnicity. Our approach in this chapter is to focus
on those interethnic relationships involving persons socially classified as belonging to different "races," although we acknowledge
that many interethnic relationships (e.g., interreligious, international) involve persons socially classified as belonging to the same
"race" (Gaines & Ickes, 1997).

this book; see also Gaines, 1995b), what common ground serves to bring together individuals differing in ethnicity? In part, we may answer that question by undercutting its logic. That is, ethnic groups do not differ in *kind* but, rather, in *degree* as far as the aforementioned values are concerned. In addition, we may point to shared cultural inheritances among the nation's minority groups (e.g., between African Americans and Puerto Ricans; between Mexican Americans and Native American; see Flores, 1985). However, it is possible to identify certain values that transcend the cultures of majority as well as minority group members.

One such value, which has been labeled variously as "feminism" (French, 1985; Gaines, 1994b), "communalism" (Gaines, 1997; Myers, 1993), and even "expressive individualism" (Bellah et al., 1985; see also Gaines, 1995b), probably is termed most accurately as *romanticism,* or an orientation toward the welfare of one's romantic relationship (Doherty, et al. 1994; Sprecher et al. 1994). In this chapter, we shall discuss the influence of romanticism on patterns of interpersonal resource exchange between persons differing in ethnicity, especially between African Americans and Anglos. Along the way, we shall argue that at least some individuals among *all* ethnic groups embrace individuals from ethnic groups different from their own, largely on the basis of a shared orientation toward their romantic relationships. We shall focus on Black male-White female relationships, owing to the intense public scrutiny that such relationships have undergone (Gaines & Ickes, 1997; Hernton, 1965). However, given that such relationships constitute only about 15% of all interracial marriages (Staples, 1994), we shall attempt to formulate hypotheses that can be applied to interethnic relationships as a whole.

Romanticism Among Members of Various Ethnic Groups

In the first *Handbook of Social Psychology,* Wallis (1935) contributed a chapter on the "Social History of the White Man." That a chapter acknowledging Anglos' ethnicity appeared in what would become a major mainstream social psychology book prior to the United States's involvement in

World War II is fascinating in itself. Interestingly, except for a series of salutations to the technological and scientific advances of Anglos (see also Cook & Kono, 1977), the tone of Wallis's chapter is strongly anti-White. Consider this excerpt from Wallis (1935):

> The white man has destroyed natural resources, mineral, vegetable, and animal, over great areas of the world; he has annihilated native peoples so ruthlessly that in many parts of the world a few hundred years, or even less than a hundred years, of contact with whites leaves no trace of the people who were occupying the soil when the whites appeared. . . . Such, essentially, is the story in every land to which the Anglo-Saxon has gone.
>
> And what, precisely, has European civilization to offer in compensation? Much, by way of science and technology; little, indeed, by way of a more satisfying scheme of social life than is known to other peoples. The material conditions of life in Western civilization have been greatly improved. And yet it is difficult to be sure that on the whole Western civilization has increased the comfort or the satisfaction of living. This in spite of its creation of material comforts and of spiritual satisfactions which in themselves seem to enhance life. Leonardo da Vinci had in mind the white man when he said: "The works of men's hands will become the cause of their death." (pp. 358–359)

If Wallis (1935) was correct in assessing the nature of interethnic behavior on the part of Anglos, can we assume that interethnic relationships are doomed to conflict and strife, exploitation and injustice? Some social scientists might be willing to make just such a case. After all, the legacy of slavery tells us that many White men felt they could force sex upon African American women with impunity (Rosenblatt, Karis, & Powell, 1995). Similarly, the legacy of colonization is such that scores of fortune seekers from Spain not only plundered Native American treasures but placed native females (whether at the "age of consent" or not) into concubinage (Sanjek, 1994). In fact, the majority of African Americans and Latinas/os in the United States carry these legacies in their genes as the byproducts of "race mixing" (Porterfield, 1978; Root, 1992).

Interethnic marriages are, on average, less stable that intraethnic marriages (Heer, 1974; but see also Gaines & Ickes, 1997). Taking intergroup conflict at face value, the relative instability of interethnic marriages may not be surprising. Together with the propensity for parents (regardless of ethnicity) to steer their offspring toward mates having similar educational, religious, and "racial" characteristics (Gaines & Ickes, 1997; Goode, 1959), the prospects for endurance of Black-White and other interethnic marriages would appear to be slim at best. Perhaps this is one reason why interracial marriages—more than 70% of which involve Anglos paired with Asian Americans or with Latinas/os (Sanjek, 1994)—constitute only about 3% of all marriages in the United States (Gaines & Ickes, 1997).

Nonetheless, some men and women do choose to cross the "color line." Against tremendous odds, some of these interethnic marriages do stand the test of time. Furthermore, interethnic marriages are not inherently asymmetrical in terms of power, contrary to what some social scientists and laypersons often believe (Baber, 1937; Porterfield, 1978; Rosenblatt et al. 1995). On what basis do these men and women decide that they will enter into matrimony, knowing that American society still is relatively intolerant of such unions?

Ultimately, the act of crossing the color line via marriage represents a personal choice that partners must affirm continuously in the face of racist reactions from strangers, acquaintances, and even family members (Gaines & Ickes, 1997; Rosenblatt et al. 1995). To outside observers, such a choice might seem naive at best. After all, even if love is color-blind, the harsh realities of prejudice and discrimination undoubtedly place interethnic relationships under an uncomfortable spotlight (see Allport, 1954). However, the humanistic psychological perspective of Carl Rogers (1961, 1972) suggests that individuals who exercise their free will and select marriage partners as a matter of personal choice might be *less* susceptible to identity confusion than are those individuals who feel constrained to marry within their own ethnic group (Nye, 1986).

Rogers probably is best known for his concept of *unconditional positive regard*, which is the process by which an individual demonstrates affection and respect toward another person without any strings attached (Bischof, 1964; Ewen, 1993; Nye, 1986). It is no accident that in comparing the stances of psychoanalytic, behaviorist, and humanistic therapies toward their clients, Foa and Foa (1974) concluded that only humanistic therapists were likely to respond to clients' revelations by giving affection and respect. (Psychoanalysts presumably *deny* affection and respect, whereas behaviorists presumably do not offer such intangible resources to their clients.) Rogers's own efforts at resolving tensions between Black and White South Africans testifies to his conviction that interethnic conflict is not inevitable (see also Gaines & Reed, 1994, 1995) and can be overcome at the interpersonal level.

Rogers's conceptualization of unconditional positive regard within the context of one-on-one relationships is compatible with the value orientation of *romanticism*, a constellation of beliefs, including "love at first sight, there is only one true love, true love lasts forever, . . . and love can overcome any obstacles" (Sprecher et al., 1994, p. 353). The results of a variety of empirical studies (e.g., Doherty et al., 1994; Fehr, 1994; Sprecher et al., 1994) indicate that romanticism is embraced by at least some individuals within every major ethnic group. Indeed, romanticism may be *especially* prominent in interactive relationships because those relationships often do not benefit from the sources of social support (e.g., family and friends) that partners in intraethnic relationships typically take for granted. Hence, partners in interethnic relationships often find that their only reliable sources of love and esteem are each other.

Consistent with this perspective is the qualitative finding (e.g., Porterfield, 1978; Rosenblatt et al. 1995) that partners in interethnic relationships often discover that their jointly held beliefs about love conquering all are essential in sustaining them through social situations in which they face hostility from strangers, acquaintances, friends, and family. On the basis of qualitative data, then, romantic love appears to fuel interethnic couples' resolve to marry (Baber, 1937; Crohn, 1995; Porterfield, 1978; Rosenblatt et al. 1995). More precisely, we may hypothesize that the individuals who make up those interethnic couples who do persevere have highly developed capacities for giving affection and respect, for attending to each other's needs for socioemotional intimacy. Baber's

(1937) pre-World War II research on mixed marriages—conducted three decades before the United States Supreme Court declared all state anti-miscegenation laws unconstitutional (Spickard, 1989)—lends support to such a hypothesis.

On the one hand, we would not conclude (as some researchers have done; see Stephan & Stephan, 1989) that interethnic marriages necessarily have rendered ethnic ingroup-outgroup distinctions increasingly obscure. On the other hand, we are not baffled (as some researchers seem to be; see Aldridge, 1973) that the rate of intermarriage has increased steadily since World War II (Tucker & Mitchell-Kernan, 1990) despite the surge in ethnic consciousness among members of ethnic minorities in the United States (and, we might add, among some Anglos; see Alba & Chamlin, 1983). If we acknowledge that romantic love forms a major part of the socioemotional foundation for marriage in general (Fehr, 1993, 1994), then we would not expect the interpersonal "rules of the game" to change when we shift from intraethnic to interethnic relationship contexts.

Stereotypes: Depraved Men

As has been noted earlier, when Black men are discussed in connection with Black women, those men frequently are portrayed as "spineless" or as "weak" in both popular and scientific accounts. However, when Black men are associated in some way with *White* women, those men are transformed—through the magic of stereotyping—into "brutes." Just as Dr. Jeckyl's fateful encounter with a dangerous chemical brew converted him from a mild-mannered fellow into the notorious Mr. Hyde, presumably all that is needed in order to change African American men from lambs into lions is the elixir known as White female charm. Though such descriptions may seem like wild exaggerations of the discrepant ways in which Black men are characterized in scientific and lay accounts, such descriptions continue to exemplify the contradictory yet self-perpetuating nature of racial stereotypes regarding Black men in America.

Throughout the twentieth century, some writers on interethnic relations have been overtly racist and seem to have prided themselves on their unscientific rationales. For example, in *White Women, Coloured Men*, Champly (1939) used the term "darkies" at will when referring to African American men. Predictably, Champly depicted the issue of "miscegenation" as one of men of color across the globe coveting women of European descent. Moreover, Champly (1939) maintained that the animalistic nature of Black men served at once to captivate and shackle unwitting White women.

In Champly's opinion, Black men do not "court" White women. On the contrary, Black men ostensibly overpower White women—if not by sheer muscular strength, then by an irresistibly primitive scent that they emit! Whether Black men possess the mental capacity required to engage in romantic (as opposed to lewd) dialogue with White women is at most questionable in the interpersonal world constructed by Champly. Apparently, in such an interpersonal world, Black men compensate for their lack of verbal prowess by resorting to hormonal secretions and aggressive seduction.

Why were African American and other "coloured" men so attracted to European American and other "White" women? The answer to this question, in the mind of Champly (1939), is twofold. First, African American and other females of color might be seen as women but never as *ladies*. Black women, according to Champly, inevitably represented pale imitations (pun intended) of "true" womanhood. That is, in the United States and around the world, Black women and other women of color supposedly envied the magnificent beauty of White women. As a result, Champly (1939) believed, African American and other "coloured" women tried to mimic women of European descent through exaggerated styles of dress, mannerisms, and attempts at attaining the finer things in life. Try as they might, alas, Black women were incapable of achieving "femininity" in its essence. Thus, Champly (1939) argued, Black men (who, despite their shortcomings as rational beings, apparently knew the difference between "fool's gold" and "the real thing" when they saw it) could not help but seek greener or, more accurately, *whiter* romantic pastures.

White women, on the other hand, had developed "femininity" into an art form. Champly (1939) asserted that the White woman was "the most beautiful thing we can imagine" (p. 199). While White men busied themselves with the mundane concerns of day-to-day, dog-eat-dog survival, White women "have soaked themselves in scented baths until they have made themselves anaemic, hyper-sensitive, super-effeminate" (p. 213). Champly went on to warn White men that they were letting "their" women fall prey to unscrupulous Black men. In fact, Champly (1939) saw the White man's interpersonal burden as a moral imperative; White men must enter competition in earnest for the sexual, if not emotional, affection of White women. After all, complained Champly, "coloured" men had discovered the pleasures of White women in all sections of the globe. As Champly (1939) saw it, the darker-hued men of this planet were practicing reverse colonization by debauching White women and shaming White men.

Other writers on the subject of Black-White sex and marriage have been equally subjective in their racism. For example, in *What Price Integration?* (1956), A. E. Burgess confessed, "Now, I do not claim to be a scientist, nor do I have a great amount of original data to contribute to this discussion" (p. 42). Nevertheless, Burgess's lack of scientific expertise did not dissuade him from attacking integration in general and interethnic marriage in particular with pseudoscientific appeals to readers.

Burgess contended that African Americans were biologically inferior to Anglos and that the "American way" was threatened by communist-inspired rabble-rousers pushing for full inclusion of Blacks in American society. Burgess even went so far as to remove from their original context some quotes by the renowned African American scholar-activist, W.E.B. Du Bois, in such a way that Du Bois's spirited assaults against racism (Gaines & Reed, 1994, 1995) were reconstructed as "tacit acceptance" of the inherent superiority of White over Black blood! And, in one of those curious feats of logistic gymnastics that so often characterizes anti-miscegenation writings, Burgess hypothesized that Blacks and Whites naturally despise each other, yet only concerted resistance on the part of red-blooded, American White men could keep the two "races" from mingling: "What I am arguing against is *social equality* between Negroes and whites. Social equality leads to intermarriage, as surely as night follows day, and unrestricted marriage between the two races would be a calamity for the white race" (p. 86, emphasis in the original).

Still other commentators on "intermarriage" seemingly

have repudiated racist scientific and lay sentiments of the past but actually have proceeded to offer variants on the same theme of intolerance. For example, in *Sexual Racism*, Stember correctly noted that the type of miscegenation that elicited the most passionate reprisals from the White-dominated society was that of the Black male-White female variety. Moreover, Stember (1976) observed that even in the post-Civil Rights era, some White supremacists attempted to capitalize on latent sexual-racial fears among Anglos by depicting Black male-White female relationships in a stereotypical manner: "The male is treated as a kind of animal-like creature, placed in juxtaposition with a frail, slender, usually blond white girl" (p. 22).

Unfortunately, Stember's efforts to educate academicians and laypersons alike vis-à-vis the prevalence of racist portrayals of interethnic sex and marriage ultimately fall short. Like many other writers past and present, Stember failed to acknowledge that mutual affection and respect can provide a basis for solidarity in Black-White romantic relationships. Moreover, Stember reduced Black-White attraction to eroticism.

Few social scientists have tackled the issue of interethnic romance as forthrightly as has Gordon Allport. Allport's classic *The Nature of Prejudice* (1954) still stands as an influential work several decades after its initial publication (Gaines & Reed, 1994, 1995). Allport maintained that many Anglos associated sexuality with African Americans (particularly with African American men) because of their own inability to reconcile sexual urges within themselves (whether directed specifically toward African Americans or not). Though Stember undoubtedly would take Allport to task for explaining American society's taboos against interethnic sex and marriage in psychoanalytic terms, Allport (unlike Stember) was unflinching in denouncing the sexist and racist stereotypes that not only curbed intermarriage but served to "keep Negroes in their place" generally.

Oddly enough, the most vociferous attacks on "race mixing" generally have come from the one region of the country in which White male-Black female marriage traditionally outpaced Black male-White female marriage in sheer numbers: the South (Spickard, 1989). Thus, Allport's psychoanalytically oriented account of Anglos' resistance to interethnic sex and marriage does seem plausible when one realizes that certain Southern White men have been especially likely to protest against *those interethnic relationships that do not include White men.*

As it turns out, even Allport (1954) was not free entirely as far as stereotypes were concerned. In a footnote (p. 381), he hinted that "evidence" of African American males' inefficacy in intraethnic home settings (i.e., the stereotype of the effeminate male, as has been discussed earlier in this volume) argued against bigots' fantasies of African American men as sexual threats (i.e., the stereotype of the depraved male described in the present chapter). Nevertheless, Allport clearly believed that White males' fears regarding the wanton sexuality of Black men basically were unfounded.

Part of the reason why the issue of Black male sexual aggression toward White women remains cloudy, both in academia and in the larger social sphere, is that a segment of the African American community evidently has accepted the stereotyped image (Awkward, 1995). In 1991, filmmaker Spike Lee's *Jungle Fever* caused a commotion upon its release because its primary subject matter was an interethnic affair between an African American man and an Italian American woman. In *Jungle Fever*, the African American man's proclaimed motivation for pursuing that illicit relationship was curiosity. However, it is noteworthy that the Italian American woman's motivation was *not* easily dismissed as submission to Black animalism.

Similarly, in *Another Country*, novelist James Baldwin (1963) invites the reader to witness the unfolding of a relationship between an angry Black Northerner, Rufus, and a pitiable White Southerner, Leona, from its lust-ridden beginning to its abuse-ridden ending—all during the first quarter of the novel! From the tone of *Another Country*, it is obvious that Baldwin is attempting to challenge racist and sexist stereotypes by pairing Rufus and Leona. Yet the manner in which Baldwin brings Rufus and Leona together—at a party where alcohol and marijuana help supply the "ambiance" (such as it is)—undermines Baldwin's own intentions. The implication seems to be that if it weren't for the drugs, a "rational" Rufus and Leona might not even find each other attractive and they certainly would not act on whatever attraction they did feel toward each other.

The societal stereotype of African American men as would-be sexual assailants abounds in common folklore and in academic treatises. Many societal institutions have conveyed the message that "race mixing"—especially with African American men and Anglo women—is not only wrong but could prove deadly to the participants. Relatively few African Americans ever have supported laws banning interethnic marriage or sex (National Research Council, 1989). Nevertheless, relatively few have *advocated* "race mixing" as prudent or wise. In fact, some Black nationalists have rivaled White segregationists in the fervor with which they have denounced interethnic romance (Porterfield, 1978; Rosenblatt et al. 1995; Spickard, 1989).

So far, we have limited our attention to the so-called "depravity" of the men (in particular, Black men) who pursue interethnic romantic relationships. But what about the "accessibility" of the women (in particular, White women) who join in these unconventional romances? In the next section, we shall give equal time to common perceptions, stereotyped though they may be, regarding women in interethnic relationships.

Stereotypes: Accessible Women

In 1951, Morton Deutsch and Mary Evans Collins published a landmark study on interracial housing projects. Deutsch and Collins found that, contrary to then-popular opinion, integrated housing projects did *not* trigger "race wars" but, over time, actually ameliorated whatever tensions between Black and White tenants had existed initially. Even more intriguing was the revelation that interracial housing promoted friendlier intraethnic *and* interethnic relations than did segregated biracial housing (i.e., with Blacks occupying one section and Whites occupying the other section of the complex). However, some of the White homemakers in integrated projects expressed apprehension over the possibility that their children's (especially their daughters') social relationships with neighboring Black children had become *too* friendly (cf. Allport, 1954).

Why has the specter of interethnic romance been raised so often when the females potentially involved are White? Part of the answer lies in the attitude, expressed by Champly and discussed in the preceding section, that White womanhood is a veritable work of art. Indeed, Champly referred to White womanhood as "our greatest sin." That is, European culture had produced a creature so remarkable that *all* men, even those of the "mongrel races," were compelled to seek her out.

Another, and perhaps more important, reason why many Whites have been alarmed over the possibility that their sisters and daughters, wives and mothers might enter into personal relationships with men of color (in particular, Black men) is that, in some circles, White women have been perceived as too weak to resist the advances of "mongrels." Champly (1939) made this point explicit by asking rhetorically, "How many white women . . . do not deliberately make mixed marriages, but are driven into them: victims who live in terror, perhaps in despair?" (p. 239). Again, the thought that some White women choose willingly to date and marry men of color seems too fantastic for Champly to entertain.

If we accept the premise (see R. Collins, 1989) that women traditionally have been expected to act as sexual gatekeepers, it is not hard to understand why some Whites have fostered the belief that White women in interethnic romantic relationships have been victimized: *They must have been overpowered. Or, someone must have stolen the key.* The alternative would be to admit that whatever attraction existed was mutual, that true romance had blossomed, and that sexual intercourse was not forced but instead evolved as a natural consequence of emotional intimacy.

Champly and others of similar ideological persuasion have, at times, acknowledged that White women were worthy of affection and respect and were accorded such by men of color. However, those ideologues also have assumed that men of color primarily viewed White women contemptuously, as if men of color were saying, "You are unable to defend yourself against me. How can I regard you as anything other than a prize to be possessed?" It is as if Champly and others have been determined to reduce interpersonal resource exchange to sexual bartering, rather than the reciprocal giving of affection and respect that Foa and Foa (1974) viewed as a vital part of what separated personal from impersonal relationships as a whole.

Given that most discussions of interethnic romance have been limited to the allegedly insatiable desire of African American men for Anglo women, to what degree have Anglo women either rebuked or internalized societal stereotypes about themselves as vulnerable to the advances of African American men? Allport (1954) maintained that White women (1) secretly wanted physical, if not emotional, intimacy with Black men and (2) accepted the dual stereotypes of Black men as depraved and themselves as reluctantly accessible because the stereotypes helped preserve their own stereotypically virtuous image.

Allport's (1954) perspective on Anglo women and interethnic personal relationships was not unique. Allport merely shifted the blame for libidinous desire from Black men to White women. Conspicuous in its absence is the acknowledgment, by Allport or by many other writers regarding interethnic romance, that individuals' need for affection and respect not only can transcend the presumed boundaries of ethnicity but also may overshadow eroticism in interethnic and intraethnic relationships alike.

The elevation of mythology to the status of social-scientific "fact" was not merely a phenomenon unique to Allport or other White scholars, however. Consider African American scholar Calvin Hernton's *Sex and Racism in America* (1965). Hernton argued that, although the myth of White womanhood was invented and propagated primarily by Southern White men, both Black men *and* White women embraced that myth so thoroughly that they were tormented mutually by carnal thoughts regarding interethnic encounters. According to Hernton, Anglo women were idealized to the point that, in order to live up to the high ideals (e.g., chastity, lack of libido) each of them "had to deny and purge herself of every honest and authentic female emotion that is vital to being a healthy woman" (p. 15). Left atop her pedestal by the White man (who presumably sought sexual gratification in the arms of the Black woman) and feeling lonely, Hernton would have us believe, the White woman became fixated on the forbidden entity, the Black man.

At times, Hernton (1965) seemed ambivalent regarding his own statements about sexuality and ethnicity. For instance, Hernton was reluctant to give the benefit of the doubt to those Anglo women whom he interviewed. Even though most of those women stated that altruistic love was their primary motivation for persevering in interethnic personal relationships, Hernton assumed that the women were hiding their "real" desire, namely, sex. Nevertheless, Hernton (1965) asserted that "because of what we *think*, because of an *abnormal* society . . . the very hostilities of the outside world sometimes tend to weld together, in love and compatibility, a white woman and a black man more tenaciously than most of us are wont to surmise" (p. 54). Hernton apparently realized that interethnic romance could not be reduced to sexual mechanics yet seemed uncomfortable with such a realization.

Hernton's analysis of interethnic relationships raises interesting questions about the thoughts, feelings, and actions of those Anglo women who are partners in such relationships. For instance, how do individual White women come to terms with the sexist/racist belief that if they marry "outside their race" they must be promiscuous (not only when interacting with Black men but with White men as well)? How do those women deal with ostracism from their own families? Furthermore, how do they react to the stereotypical assumption that they are not competent enough to *choose* their marriage partners but simply are "giving in" to Black men's desires? Unfortunately, Hernton's (1965) work does not offer answers to those questions.

All too often, social scientists and laypersons alike fail to acknowledge that many Anglo women consciously and willingly marry African American men and other men of color. This apparent blindness to the social-psychological experiences of White women in interethnic relationships often is reflected and perpetuated by American mass media. Take, for instance, the motion picture *Guess Who's Coming to Dinner*, which was quite provocative upon its release in the late 1960s. Even though the film broke new ground by depicting interethnic romance between a White woman and a Black man, the focal point of the film was not the thoughts or feelings of the White fiancee but, instead, the reaction of her father.

Another example of conventionality in media depictions of White women's encounters with Black men may be found in Marilyn French's (1977) novel *The Women's Room*. In the novel, the most salient African American male character (Mick) is introduced as a rapist; his victim (Chris) is a college student and daughter of one of the protagonists (Val). Clearly, French (1977) is attempting to demonstrate the extent to which racism is institutionalized (e.g., in the legal and judicial systems). Ironically, racism is emphasized *within the context of forced sex with a Black male as instigator and a White female as unwitting victim.* Furthermore, French manages to invoke the image of the overbearing Black matriarch (as was described earlier in this volume) between episodes of sexual violence.

Before moving on, we hasten to add that just as Black male-White female relationships have been stereotyped as to the intrusiveness of men and the defenselessness of women in interethnic personal relationships, so too have White male-Black female relationships—to a degree. In condemning White rape of Black women from the slavery era to the present, scientific and lay writers alike have left the impression that conflict is inevitable in interethnic relationships. Black women have been cast as aggressors more often than White women in the popular imagination (Hernton, 1965). Nevertheless, African American and Anglo women alike have been depicted as victims for the most part.

This is not to deny the prevalence of victimization of women (especially African American women) in interethnic relationships. However, we cannot assume that aggression against women is to be found solely or even primarily in interethnic relationships, nor can we assume that aggression against women necessarily is the norm in interethnic relationships. As Johnston (1939) mused, "Of only one thing can we be reasonably certain; miscegenation is a normal consequence of human beings living and working together at common tasks. No unusual moral qualities, on the part of either group, needs to be assumed" (p. 1).

Theoretical Perspectives on Interethnic Relationships

Throughout this chapter, we have alluded to the influence that Freudian psychoanalytic theory has had upon scientific and lay perceptions of partners in interethnic marriages and opponents of interethnic marriage. We noted that Allport (1954), for example, interpreted American society's aversions to "miscegenation" and "intermarriage" as the result of many Whites' repression of their own interethnic desires and subsequent projection of those desires onto Blacks. Also, as we have observed, Hernton (1965) argued that Blacks and Whites alike, whether male or female, were obsessed with interethnic sexuality. But what did Freud himself have to say about the matter?

In *Totem and Taboo*, Freud (1918/1946) proposed a "racial psychology" that on the surface might seem amenable to the study of interethnic relationships. Unfortunately, Freud's racial psychology presupposes a hierarchy of "superior" and "inferior" races in which Europeans and European Americans inevitably wind up on top. Freud (1918/1946) suggested that exogamy (i.e., sex or marriage between persons belonging to different socially defined groups; Kephart & Jedlicka, 1988) was practiced widely among "primitive" races because such races held the superstitious belief that physical intimacy between members of the same tribe automatically constituted incest. In contrast, Freud maintained, the "advanced" races were not consumed with such a fear and, therefore, could practice endogamous (i.e., within-group) sex and marriage freely.

Could Freud's speculations regarding exogamy as the norm among "inferior" races and of endogamy as the norm among "superior" races possibly have found favor in the literature on interethnic relationships? Apparently so, judging from the writings of overt racists such as Champly (1939) and from the works of respected social scientists (e.g., Reuter, 1918) who were not blatantly racist yet maintained that persons of color wanted to mate with Anglos (but not vice versa). In any event, Freud seemed to be preoccupied with *totemism*, a socioreligious practice in which "backward" ethnic groups supposedly "come to select the names of animals, plants and inanimate objects for themselves and their tribes" (p. 142) and in which *"the members of the same totem are not allowed to enter into sexual relations with each other; that is, they cannot marry each other"* (p. 7, emphasis in the original). Freud even maintained that the phenomenon of fictive kinship (e.g., referring to nonbiological ingroup members as "sister" or "brother") was evidence of totemism. In turn, totemism was a cultural manifestation of the Oedipus complex that, presumably, each tribe member unsuccessfully sought to resolve.

Of course, no Freudian analysis would be complete without at least a passing reference to the "weakness" of women (see French, 1985, for a critique of psychoanalysis and feminism). Freud did not undertake to verify his hypotheses via firsthand observation of "primitive" races (which he placed within Australia, America, and Africa). Instead, Freud relied heavily upon a few anthropological accounts and interpreted those accounts within the confines of psychoanalytic theory. At any rate, Freud did not let his lack of experience with so-called practitioners of totemism stop him from blaming pregnant women for the practice.

In response to Freud's conceptual assault on pregnant women as the would-be "mothers" of totemism, Karen Horney (1967) might have suspected Freud of "pregnancy envy." Of all the neo-Freudian theorists, Horney challenged Freud's views on femininity most decisively (Hall & Lindzey, 1970). Horney's volume of compiled works, *Feminine Psychology* (1967), refutes many of Freud's central hypotheses regarding gender and personality. How, then, would Horney's neo-Freudian psychology deal with Freud's racial psychology?

Concerning interethnic relationships, Horney asserted that in the long run, sexual obsession in itself is not sufficient to maintain marital satisfaction. In interethnic and intraethnic marital relationships alike, the key to satisfaction and stability is individuals' realization that they cannot expect to receive affection and respect consistently without giving those interpersonal resources in return. Furthermore, Horney believed, individuals must accept their partners' imperfections to a greater degree and acknowledge their own imperfections more often than they have been socialized to acknowledge. Horney's perspective on mutual acceptance in interethnic relationships is similar in many ways to that articulated by Rogers.

Horney also did not accept the premise that sexual relations were destined to take the dual forms of male gratification and female passivity. For one thing, female sexuality had to be taken into account; Freud and other "masculinist" psychoanalysts were too willing to deny—or, alternatively, to deride—eroticism among women. In addition, Horney believed that the concept of "recreational sex" (i.e., sexuality outside the context of a loving, supportive relationship) inevitably was male-biased because for most women, the potential consequences of sex, particularly pregnancy, were too real to be trivialized in such a manner. Thus, Horney's account of gender and personal relationships provides us with several grounds on which to reject the myth of interethnic relationships as based upon male sexual aggressiveness and female acquiescence (see Ramirez, 1991).

It must be noted that Horney's neo-Freudian framework remains open to criticism. Horney, like Freud, spent an inordinate amount of time discussing the "problem" of homosexuality and searching for evidence, however elusive, as to Oedipal conflict in both men and women. Furthermore, as Hall and Lindzey (1970) pointed out, Horney agreed with Freud in several instances (e.g., regarding "castration anxiety" in females), leading some critics to ask whether Horney's theory really constituted a significant departure from Freud's.

Nevertheless, Horney's (1967) social-psychological theory of personality argued against popularly held and scientifically reified views regarding gender and ethnicity. Interestingly, according to Horney, interethnic relationships were not problematic in and of themselves. Rather, conflict in those relationships might be expected to ensue to the extent that interethnic spouses themselves internalized negative stereotypes regarding their partners' gender and ethnicity.

At this juncture, we may form reasoned hypotheses as to the extent to which affection and respect are displayed by men and women in interethnic heterosexual relationships, using stereotypical and romantic perspectives on interethnic relationships. In the stereotyped model, interethnic relationships are assumed to operate such that any affectionate or respectful behaviors initiated by men are likely to be reciprocated by women. However, affectionate or respectful behaviors initiated by women are *not* likely to be reciprocated by men. The stereotyped model of interpersonal resource exchange among interethnic heterosexual couples is presented in Figure 5.1. (Note the similarity between Figure 5.1 and Figure 3.1, presented earlier.)

In contrast, the romantic model assumes that men and women alike will reciprocate affectionate and respectful behaviors initiated by their partners. Furthermore, romanticism will be reflected positively and significantly in men's and women's displays of affection and respect. The romantic model of interpersonal resource exchange among interethnic couples is presented in Figure 5.2.

How well do these divergent models explain the behavior of individuals from one ethnic group toward the opposite-

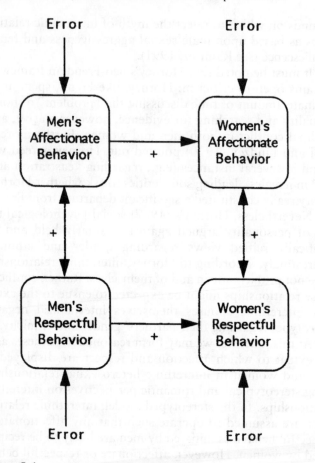

Figure 5.1:
Stereotyped model of interpersonal resource exchange among interethnic couples

gender members of another ethnic group? We shall review empirical studies concerning romanticism and interpersonal resource exchange in interethnic relationships in the next section. Unlike the previous chapters in the present volume, we will have the opportunity in this chapter to examine the results of a study (Gaines, Rios et al. 1996) specifically designed to test the viability of competing models of interpersonal resource exchange among interethnic couples.

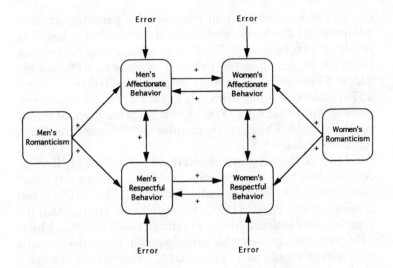

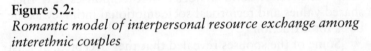

Figure 5.2:
Romantic model of interpersonal resource exchange among interethnic couples

Empirical Research on Interethnic Relationships

As we have seen, a few noteworthy studies on interethnic relationships have been conducted since the 1960s. One of the most comprehensive studies was carried out by Ernest Porterfield in 1978. Porterfield's ethnographic study included an historical overview of "miscegenation" as well as an account of more contemporary attempts by participants in the Black Power movement to curb fellow African Americans' desire for persons of the opposite gender who were not African American. Moreover, Porterfield interviewed couples in four cities (two in the North and cities in the South). All of the cities could be described as "All-American," and the majority of residents of those cities—regardless of the relative size of the Black population—generally viewed interethnic marriage with disdain.

A total of 40 couples (corresponding to roughly 60% of those initially contacted) agreed to participate in Porterfield's

111

study. The vast majority of couples who participated were composed of Black men and White women (33 couples). The resulting proportion of Black male-White female couples (83%) is higher than the national average of 67% among Black-White pairs of spouses in general (Gaines & Ickes, 1996; Gaines & Jones-Mitchell, 1996; Staples, 1994). Nevertheless, Porterfield's (1978) sample reflects the preponderance of Black male-White female couples over White male-Black female couples.

Most of the couples in Porterfield's (1978) study lived in African American communities and did not know any other interethnic couples personally. Unlike Golden (1954), but consistent with Pavela (1964), Porterfield did not find that the couples were isolated from intraethnic Black couples. Moreover, of the 80 spouses who participated in Porterfield's study, only eleven mentioned "race-related" reasons for marrying their partners. A solid majority of the spouses saw their shared values and reciprocal socioemotional intimacy as the basis for attraction.

Some of the spouses revealed that they accepted, at least in part, some of the stereotypes regarding interethnic romance (e.g., the White woman as the epitome of femininity). Nevertheless, such stereotyped views were not expressed by most of the spouses. Furthermore, according to Porterfield (1978), "A preponderance of the families reported being relatively happy. As far as marital problems are concerned, theirs are no different from those of any other marriage. Quarrels or other family disagreements seldom carry racial overtones" (p. 123).

In short, the results of Porterfield's (1978) study tend to support the romantic, rather than the stereotyped, model of socioemotional behavior in interethnic relationships. We hasten to add that Porterfield did not test resource exchange theory (Foa & Foa, 1974) directly. However, consistent with resource exchange theory, Porterfield (1978) argued that social exchange accounts casting interpersonal behavior in interethnic relationships as primarily the exchange of tangible resources (e.g., money, sex) were insufficient to explain the patterns of behavior that he encountered.

A more recent study of 21 Black/White couples in the Minneapolis/St. Paul area was published in 1995 by Paul Rosenblatt, Terri Karis, and Richard Powell. Rosenblatt, Karis, and Powell reiterated many of the points that Porterfield had made nearly twenty years earlier. However, Rosenblatt, Karis, and Powell also raised several novel issues of their own.

Rosenblatt, Karis, and Powell noted that much of the opposition of White family members to interracial marriage involves a concern that their families will lose whatever privileges accompany all-White status (see also Zack, 1993). In addition, Rosenblatt and his colleagues pointed out that even though Black family members' opposition to interracial marriage tends to be substantially less virulent than does that of White family members, the opposition that surfaces among Black and White family members alike seems more likely to be directed toward controlling the behavior of their daughters than of their sons. Perhaps most poignant, though, was the finding that in many instances, only after they married interracially did White spouses begin to understand the depth and breadth of racism that their Black partners had battled their entire lives (see also Goffman, 1963). Although Rosenblatt, Karis, and Powell (1995) were careful not to overgeneralize the results of their qualitative study, their results clearly were consistent with those reported by Porterfield (1978).

Still another study that is at least tangentially related to our discussion of affectionate and respectful behavior in interethnic relationships is the technical report by Triandis, Weldon, and Feldman (1972), mentioned in the preceding chapter of this volume on the "subjective cultures" of Anglos and African Americans. Though Triandis, Weldon, and Feldman did not examine actual behavior (whether in personal or role relationships), their findings do help us place interethnic relationships within a larger societal context. In particular, the expressed behavioral tendencies of Anglos and African Americans toward persons of the opposite gender and ethnic group may serve to illustrate the limits of applicability of stereotyped or romantic models of interethnic socioemotional behavior.

Regarding behavioral intentions toward African American women, Anglo men were less likely to trust and give assistance than were African American men, other African American women, or Anglo women. (Trust is an important component of affectionate behavior in resource exchange theory; Foa & Foa, 1974.) Triandis, Weldon, and Feldman (1972) made an intriguing observation concerning White males' behavioral tendencies vis-à-vis Black females: "The hardcore [i.e., lower-class] whites . . . show the most unfavorable stereotypes (evaluations) and behavioral intentions (little *trust* and intention to *help*; the young men (only) are willing to *go out with* her)" (p. 40). Triandis and his colleagues concluded that because young, lower-class White males were willing to date but not risk socioemotional intimacy with African American women, those males' responses reflected an exploitative stance toward Black women.

Regarding behavioral tendencies toward Anglo women, African American men were less likely to trust and ask them for advice than were European American men. (According to resource exchange theory, asking another person for advice confers respect upon the potential adviser; Foa & Foa, 1974.) However, Black men did *not* tend to stereotype White women unfavorably. Triandis, Weldon, and Feldman (1972) suggested that many Black men might maintain social distance between themselves and White women despite the fact that they harbor no ill will toward White women. Triandis and his colleagues did not detect the exploitative orientation of Black men toward White women that had been apparent among a subsample of White men toward Black women.

Regarding behavioral intentions toward African American men, Anglo women were less likely to go out with them than were African American women. Triandis, Weldon, and Feldman noticed that Anglos in general held rather negative stereotypical views of African American men. Consistent with this observation, Anglo women were significantly more likely to stay away from African American men than were African American women.

Finally, regarding behavioral tendencies toward Anglo men, African American women were less likely to help, trust, and go out with them than were Anglo women. Triandis and his colleagues seemingly de-emphasized the differences in Black and White women's responses. For example, in interpreting the results of a four-way interaction (with ethnicity, socioeconomic status, gender, and age as predictors of displays of trust), Triandis, Weldon, and Feldman implied that social class was as influential in Anglo women's ratings as it was in African American women's ratings. However, Anglo women—regardless of their socioeconomic status—tended to trust Anglo men. Among young African American lower-class and working-class women, in contrast, trust of Anglo men was low. Moreover, though Triandis and his colleagues noted widespread anti-White-male prejudice among Blacks in general, no attempt was made to link lower-class Black women's antipathy toward White men with the earlier finding that lower-class White men were especially likely to view Black women in sexually exploitive terms.

Triandis's work on the subjective cultures of Blacks and Whites offers interesting glimpses into the links between prejudice and discrimination in American society. First of all, it is notable that Black men do not appear to be driven by the aggressive desires toward White women that many Whites (particularly the White women in Triandis's own study) attribute to them. Second, Black women (at least those occupying the lower social strata and, historically, especially vulnerable to unwanted advances from White men) seem quite justified in their distrustful stance toward White men. Perhaps the fears expressed by Du Bois (1921/1975) regarding the racial/sexual "double standard" still are rational in the decades since the 1967 Supreme Court declaration of state anti-intermarriage laws as unconstitutional—despite Du Bois's hope that the removal of those laws from the American landscape would offer greater protection to African American women.

Finally, results by Gaines, Rios, Granrose, Bledsoe, Farris, Page, and Garcia (1996) make it possible to compare the utility of the stereotyped and romantic models of interpersonal resource exchange among 112 interethnic couples (all of whom were living together at the time of the study; approximately 75% of the couples were married). Gaines and his colleagues were interested primarily in evaluating the romantic model in and of itself. However, by entering the correlation matrix from Gaines, Rios, Granrose, Bledsoe, Farris, Page, and Garcia (1996) into LISREL 7 (Joreskog & Sorbom, 1979, 1989), the authors of the present chapter were able to evaluate the statistical goodness-of-fit of the romantic model *as compared to that of the stereotyped model.*

First, let us examine the goodness-of-fit of the stereotyped model. LISREL results yield a chi-square value of 28.08, with 7 degrees of freedom ($p < .01$). In LISREL and other structural equation programs, a significant chi-square suggests that the model in question provides a fit to the data that is significantly *worse* than chance. Given that the chi-square value frequently is inflated by large sample sizes, it is also useful to examine the chi-square/degrees-of-freedom ratio as an indicator of goodness-of-fit. (The degrees of freedom are calculated independently of sample size.) Typically, a chi-square value of 2.00 or higher is considered evidence of a poor fit. The chi-square/degrees-of-freedom ratio provided by the stereotyped model (4.01), together with the chi-square value in itself, suggests that the stereotyped model does not accurately reflect the correlational data from Gaines et al. (1996).

Next, let us examine the goodness-of-fit of the romantic model. The chi-square value of 2.24 with 3 degrees of freedom (*NS*) suggests that the romantic model provides an acceptable fit to the data. That is, the error associated with the model is *not* significantly greater than chance. Furthermore, the small chi-square value associated with the romantic model indicates that sample size *per se* was not responsible for the high chi-square value associated with the stereotyped model. Generally, low chi-square/degrees-of-freedom ratios are considered desirable on structural equation analysis; however, ratios below 1.00 raise the possibility that the fit of the model is "too good to be true." Thus, the chi-square/degrees-of-freedom ratio yielded by the romantic model (i.e., 0.74) is somewhat lower than optimal. Ideally, one would want to replicate the results of the romantic model in a new sample (or, perhaps, divide the data set randomly into equal halves and fit the model simultaneously to the two subsamples) before attempting to make strong causal inferences about the model.

Nevertheless, a direct comparison of the two models indicates that the romantic model provides a significantly better fit to the data than does the stereotyped model. The loss of degrees of freedom in shifting from the stereotyped to the romantic model (–4) is more than offset by the resulting decrease in chi-square (–25.84, *p* < .01). In addition, all of the hypothesized paths and correlations shown in Figure 5.2 were positive and significant. Overall, the results of Gaines et al.'s (1996) study indicate that the stereotyped model can be rejected quite readily, whereas the romantic model performed well enough to merit further examination in future studies.

The results reported by Gaines and his colleagues (1996) indicate that patterns of interpersonal resource exchange among interethnic couples largely reflect the importance of romanticism in the lives of those couples. Such results could not be explained using a stereotyped model of personal relationship processes among interethnic couples. Gaines et al.'s results lend quantitative support to the qualitative finding (Porterfield, 1978; Rosenblatt et al. 1995) that the bonds holding Anglos and African Americans together in matrimony often prove to be exceptionally strong, as they must be in order to withstand covert as well as overt hostility from many members of the dominant society. Despite the potential for ethnic conflict regarding certain values (e.g., collectivism, individualism), certain other values (e.g., romanticism) may bridge whatever cultural gaps exist between husbands and wives. As the literature reviewed in the present chapter indicates, it is just this commonality that many scholars and laypersons have ignored when considering the viability of interethnic romance.

Summary and Conclusions

As we conclude this chapter on interethnic relationships, certain caveats are in order. Although we have focused on the implicit value judgments embedded in previous authors' accounts of interethnic relationship processes, certain value judgments of our own undoubtedly have surfaced. For example, we have implied that the exchange of intangible resources emerging as properties of relationships (e.g., affection, respect) is more important to the establishment and maintenance of interethnic relationships than is the exchange of tangible resources that individuals already possess at the time that they enter into relationships (e.g., physical attractiveness, personal income). However, none of the quantitative or qualitative studies that we cited in support of the romantic model assessed the static attributes of individuals (as opposed to dynamic properties of relationships) as predictors of relationship development. Perhaps the stereotyped model tested by Gaines, Rios, Granrose, Bledsoe, Farris, Page, and Garcia (1996) is not the only viable alternative to the romantic model after all.

In addition, our examination of interethnic relationships implies that the predictors of initial attraction are identical to the predictors of sustained success. However, we have not offered proof that this is the case. Perhaps empirical studies of

117

initial attraction among cross-sex, cross-race pairs—which are virtually nonexistent in the social psychology literature— would reveal that attraction on the basis of external rather than internal attributes is more important to the establishment of interethnic heterosexual relationships than we have acknowledged.

Finally, in focusing upon romanticism as a predictor of personal relationship processes within the United States, we may have placed unnecessary limits upon our ability to generalize to interethnic relationship processes as a whole. In many nations outside of the West (e.g., China, India), individuals simply do not choose their own marriage partners; parents make these choices on behalf of their offspring via arrangements with families of similar class or caste. By presupposing that individuals have the freedom to choose their own partners, we may have generated a model of interpersonal resource exchange that is more individualistic than we had intended.

Nevertheless, we hope that the present chapter alerts relationship scholars to some of the negative biases that continue to pervade much of the social science literature on interethnic relationships. Furthermore, we hope that this chapter encourages subsequent researchers to develop *a priori* conceptual models of interethnic relationship processes. If we have accomplished that much, we will achieved a modest level of success.

Preparation of this chapter was made possible by postdoctoral fellowships from Franklin and Marshall College (1991–92), from The University of North Carolina at Chapel Hill (1992–93), and from the Ford Foundation, and by institutional funds from Pomona College. The authors are indebted to Kelly Brennan and Steve Duck for their constructive comments on an earlier version of this chapter.

6

Toward an Inclusive Model of Cultural Value Orientations and Personal Relationship Processes Among All Couples

At the outset of this book, my colleagues and I sought the answer to a simple question: When we examine the literature on personal relationships, what predominant theme do we find regarding cultural value orientations as reflected in personal relationship processes? As the preceding five chapters attest, the answer to that question depends upon which major ethnic group is under consideration. When Anglos are the ethnic group under consideration—or when ethnicity is not explicitly acknowledged at all—one primary theme that emerges is individualism (Bellah et al., 1985; Dion & Dion, 1993; Gaines, 1995b). When African Americans are the ethnic group under consideration, one primary theme that emerges is collectivism (Asante, 1981; Gaines, 1994a, 1995b; White, 1984; White & Parham, 1990). When Latinas/os are the ethnic group under consideration, one primary theme that emerges is familism (Gaines, 1994b, 1995b; Marin & Marin, 1991; Mirande, 1977). When Asian Americans are the ethnic group under consideration, one primary theme that emerges is spiritualism (Cook & Kono, 1977; Kitano & Daniels, 1988; Min, 1995). Finally, when interethnic relationships are under consideration, a primary theme that emerges is romanticism (Gaines, Rios et al., 1996; Porterfield, 1978; Rosenblatt et al., 1995).

Taken separately, the models of culture, ethnicity, and personal relationship processes presented in Figures 1.2, 2.2, 3.2, 4.2, and 5.2 could be construed as implying that (1) no cultural value can be held by more than one ethnic group and that (2) no ethnic group can hold more than one cultural value. Indeed, much of the literature on cultural values and ethnicity would lead one to just such a conclusion (Gaines, Marelich et al., 1997). In presenting the individualistic, collectivistic, familistic, spiritualistic, and romantic models, my colleagues and I have not sought to imply such a rigid one-to-one correspondence between cultural values and ethnicity. Rather, we have attempted to cast ethnicity as a potential moderator of links between cultural value orientations and personal relationship processes.

Now that we have surveyed the literature on cultural values and personal relationship processes among each of the major ethnic groups and among interethnic couples in the United States, it is time for us to step back and ask whether a more comprehensive model might be constructed from the narrowly tailored models that we have presented so far. Figure 6.1 represents an attempt toward an inclusive model of cultural value orientations and interpersonal resource exchange that, at least in theory, can be applied to *all* heterosexual romantic relationships, regardless of the relationship partners' ethnicity. Moreover, the inclusive model shown in Figure 6.1 represents an elaboration of an earlier model that I have advanced (Gaines, 1995b) regarding individualism, collectivism, and familism together as influences on patterns of interpersonal resource exchange.

Using structural equation analyses (see Loehlin, 1992; Long, 1983a, b) as well as other multivariate statistical analyses, enterprising researchers could test the statistical goodness-of-fit of the inclusive model versus the goodness-of-fit of the more narrowly focused models from the preceding five chapters in this volume, as applied to a particular sample of Anglo, African American, Latina/o, Asian American, or interethnic couples. In a variation on this strategy, Gaines, Rios, Granrose, Bledsoe, Farris, Page, and Garcia (1996) used multivariate multiple regression analyses to determine whether individualism, collectivism, and familism together explained significant variance in heterosexual interethnic relationship partners' mutual displays of affection and respect, after tak-

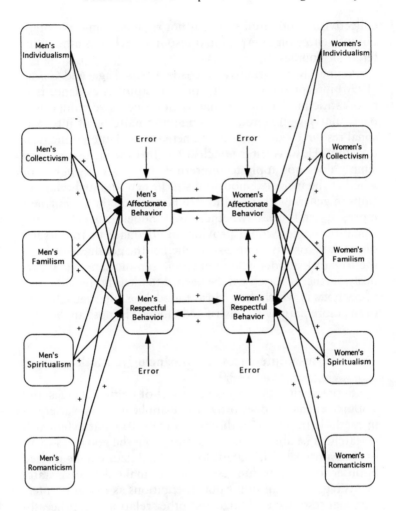

Figure 6.1:
*Inclusive model of cultural value orientations and inter-
personal resource exchange among heterosexual couples
in general*

ing the influence of romanticism into account. (Gaines et al.
[1996] did not include a measure of spiritualism in their
study.) Gaines et al. found that, prior to testing the romanticism model formally via structural equation analysis, hierarchical regressions allowed them to rule out individualism,

collectivism, and familism—but not romanticism—as potential influences on interpersonal resource exchange among interethnic couples.

Gaines, Rios, Granrose, Bledsoe, Farris, Page, and Garcia (1996) interpreted the results of their study as evidence that a romantic model, rather than a more inclusive model, was particularly well-suited for explaining patterns of interpersonal resource exchange among heterosexual interethnic relationships. However, it is not clear whether the inclusive model simply does not apply to interethnic relationships *per se* or whether the inclusive model fails to fit heterosexual relationships in general (whether interethnic or intraethnic). Furthermore, it isn't clear whether any model other than the romantic model would provide an adequate fit to correlational data for *any* sample—or whether the goodness-of-fit of the romantic model is limited to interethnic samples. Obviously, further research will be needed to identify the full range of contexts in which the inclusive model (or, alternatively, any of the more narrowly constructed models) is most applicable.

Causal Inferences and the Inclusive Model

Suppose that the inclusive model of cultural values and resource exchange does prove to be applicable to a variety of intraethnic (if not interethnic) contexts. To what extent will researchers be able to infer causality from the goodness-of-fit of such a model? Ultimately, longitudinal data will be needed in order for relationship researchers to make definitive statements regarding cultural value orientations as *causes* of interpersonal resource exchange and other relationship processes (Kenny, 1979; see also Sobel, 1995). As it stands, the one-shot nature of studies such as that conducted by Gaines, Rios, Granrose, Bledsoe, Farris, Page, and Garcia (1996) will tell us more about those models that can be disconfirmed than about those models that can be confirmed.

Given that the correlations between scores on personality questionnaires and scores on social behavior questionnaires at any one time are subject to inflation because of method variance (Kenny, 1979; Sobel, 1995), the one-shot study of interethnic relationships by Gaines et al. (1996) does not bode well for the inclusive model. Gaines and his colleagues attempted to minimize the impact of method variance on correlations between individuals' cultural values and individuals' own behavior by asking individuals to report their own cultural values but to report their *partners'* displays of affection and respect during the two weeks prior to participation in the study. In fact, even after controlling statistically for correlations between individuals' reports of their own cultural values and of their partners' interpersonal behavior, the paths from individuals' self-reported values and individuals' behavior (as reported by their partners), remained positive and significant. Nevertheless, the observed correlations between individuals' cultural values and individuals' interpersonal behavior probably represent an upper limit on the "true" correlations that are likely to be found in longitudinal research on interethnic couples. How likely is it, then, that individualism, collectivism, or familism will explain significant variance in interethnic relationship partners' displays of affection or respect in future longitudinal studies of this type?

Perhaps the most effective way to test the inclusive model, along with competing models, will be for researchers to carry out longitudinal studies of large samples (i.e., 100 or more couples) of multiple ethnic pairings. Subsequently, a multiple-group test of the inclusive model can be conducted via LISREL (Joreskog & Sorbom, 1979, 1989) or some other structural equation program. The resulting structural equation analyses will maximize the available degrees of freedom, and the goodness-of-fit of such a model that is constrained to yield identical path and correlation values across all samples (i.e., an "equal variance" model) can be compared with the goodness-of-fit of an alternative model in which all paths and correlations are allowed to vary from sample to sample (i.e., an "unequal-variance" model). If the unequal-variance model—which necessarily will entail a loss in degrees of freedom—fails to provide a significantly better fit to the correlational data than does the more parsimonious equal-variance model, then one can conclude that the inclusive model accurately reflects the "true" causal relations among the personality and social behavior variables in question.

In order to minimize the loss of degrees of freedom in shifting from the original inclusive model to an alternative model, one might wish to use modification indices (Joreskog & Sorbom, 1989) to identify specific path or correlation coefficients in specific samples that, when allowed to vary, are most likely to result in an alternative model with a significantly better fit than that provided by the original inclusive model. The disadvantage to this latter strategy is that it forces researchers to shift from a confirmatory mode to an exploratory model of causal analysis. That is, any resulting differences in goodness-of-fit between the competing models would have to be replicated in *a priori* tests before one could retain or discard the original inclusive model.

In any event, my collaborators and I hope that the inclusive model will be tested, along with competing models, by researchers who are interested in the myriad of potential cultural and ethnic influences on personal relationship processes. Researchers could, for example, go beyond the results of the research conducted on interethnic relationships in the study by Gaines, Rios, et al. (1996) and ask whether the inclusive model fits all gender-ethnic pairings equally well. For example, Gaines et al. (1996) did not collect sufficient data to determine whether the inclusive model fits correlational data for Anglo male-Black female pairs better than it fits correlational data for Latino male-Anglo female pairs, or vice versa. Above all else, we hope that the inclusive model and other models presented in this volume will encourage personal relationship scholars to propose and test theory-driven models of culture, ethnicity, and personal relationship processes.

Comparing Culturally Deficient and Culturally Sensitive Models: Fair Tests or Straw Theories?

In Chapters 2 through 5 of this volume, my collaborators and I have depicted culturally sensitive models of interpersonal resource exchange as capable of explaining significantly greater variance in relationship partners' behavior than can stereotyped or culturally deficient models. In the previous chapter, we presented secondary analyses of data collected initially by Gaines, Rios, Granrose, Bledsoe, Farris, Page, and Garcia (1996) and concluded that the romantic model (See Figure 5.2) provided a significantly better fit to the correlational data than did the stereotyped model (Figure 5.1). However, it is possible that we have stacked the deck by proposing stereotyped models that are methodologically as well as culturally deficient. Have we merely invented straw theories, labeled conveniently as stereotyped models, that could not be empirically supported even if a grain of truth (Allport, 1954) were to apply to the ethnic groups in question?

Conceptually speaking, my colleagues and I did not really invent the stereotyped models depicted in the preceding four chapters. As numerous reviews of the literature on culture, ethnicity, and individual well-being have shown (e.g., Carter, 1995; Chin, 1994; Comas-Diaz, 1994; Helms, 1990), distorted and negative assumptions regarding persons of color persist within clinical and developmental psychology. Similarly, as numerous reviews of the literature on culture, ethnicity, and interpersonal well-being have shown (e.g., Boyd-Franklin & Garcia-Preto, 1994; Gaines, 1995b; Staples & Mirande, 1980), distorted and negative assumptions about relationships involving persons of color persist within personality and social psychology. In addition, just as culturally deficient models have not yet been abandoned completely within mainstream psychology, so too have culturally sensitive models not yet taken hold (McAdoo, 1993). In the preceding four chapters of this book, my co-authors and I have attempted to describe the dynamic tension between these competing theoretical perspectives as accurately as possible.

Methodologically speaking, though, the "straw theory" hypothesis has merit. With the exception of the stereotyped model regarding Asian American relationship processes (in which neither gender's behavior is predicted to influence the other gender's behavior), the culturally deficient models postulate that covariance between men's and women's behavior reflects unidirectional causality. However, a structural equation model postulating bidirectional causality might provide a significantly better fit to the data than does the stereotyped model simply because the behavioral measures administered at any one time do not lend themselves to assumptions about who influences whom (Kenny, 1979, 1988). By collecting behavioral information at multiple times, researchers will be in a position to state conclusively whether the assumption of unidirectionality presents a statistically viable alternative to the assumption of bidirectional causality in relationship partners' behavior.

✳ Additional Covariates of Culture as Potentially Reflected in Personal Relationship Processes

By emphasizing value orientations as cultural influences on personal relationship processes, my colleagues and I have de-emphasized a host of covariates of culture that might be reflected in relationship partners' behavior. Consider the potential impact of religious denomination, social class, immigrant status, nation of origin, and age group upon patterns of interpersonal resource exchange among members of various ethnic groups (see Gallagher, 1995). It might have been interesting, for instance, if we had examined the implications of (1) a religious denomination model of resource exchange among Anglos (e.g., Jewish persons as displaying more affection and respect than do Protestants or Catholics), (2) a social-class model of resource exchange among African Americans (e.g., working-class individuals as displaying more affection and respect than do lower-class or middle-class individuals), (3) an immigrant status model among Latinas/os (e.g., first-generation Chicanas/os as displaying more affection and respect than do second-generation or third-generation Chicanas/os), (4) a nation of origin model of resource exchange among Asian Americans (e.g., Vietnamese Americans as displaying more affection or respect than do Chinese Americans or Japanese Americans), or (5) a model of resource exchange among interethnic couples of a particular age group (e.g., World War II-era individuals as displaying more affection or respect than do baby boomers or Generation X-ers). Ultimately, one could envision an inclusive model of resource exchange among all couples that takes all of the aforementioned variables into account as influences on interpersonal behavior.

Such a dramatically different way of conceptualizing the links among culture, ethnicity, and interpersonal resource exchange reveals an intriguing paradox regarding the relationship between psychologically oriented and sociologically oriented social-psychological perspectives on personal relationship processes. On the one hand, my collaborators and I have drawn heavily upon sociological studies of personal relationships involving persons of color. On the other hand, the brand of exchange theory that we have placed at the core of our models of culture, ethnicity, and personal relationship processes in this book is the psychologically oriented resource exchange theory of Foa and Foa (1974), rather than the sociologically oriented social exchange theory of Homans (1961).

The apparent paradox regarding the relative importance assigned to sociologically and psychological social psychology vis-à-vis personal relationship processes can be explained, at least in part, by taking a critical look at conceptual and methodological issues within the two social psychologies (Stephan & Stephan, 1985). Conceptually speaking, variables such as value orientations fall squarely within the domain of sociological social psychology (see Kluckhohm & Strodtbeck, 1961). Nevertheless, value orientations and social group memberships can be construed as individual-difference variables, which suggests that these variables fall within the domain of psychological social psychology (Wiggins, 1979).

Methodologically speaking, continuous predictors such as individualism, collectivism, familism, spiritualism, and romanticism are particularly amenable to the path and structural equation analyses that traditionally have been associated with sociological social psychology (Sobel, 1995). In contrast, categorical predictors such as religious denomination, social class, immigrant status, nation of origin, and age group are more amenable to the analyses of variance that have been associated with psychological social psychology (Jones, 1985). Nevertheless, because these categorical predictors are not manipulated by experimenters but instead are properties of individuals, one would be hard-pressed to portray analyses of variance involving the aforementioned social group variables as exemplars of psychologically oriented methodology.

Value orientations occupy an interesting middle ground between those variables that clearly are psychological in content (e.g., personality traits; Ewen, 1993) and those variables that clearly are sociological in content (e.g., social roles; Braithwaite & Scott, 1991). Value orientations frequently are operationalized in terms of the survey questionnaire responses favored within psychological social psychology (Harvey, Hendrick, & Tucker, 1988), yet the resulting data frequently are analyzed using the correlational methods favored within sociological social psychology (Kenny, 1988). In addition, value orientations are presumed to operate at the level of society (Kluckhohn & Strodtbeck, 1961) yet typically are measured at the level of the individual (Gelfand, Triandis, & Chan,

1996). By measuring cultural value orientations at the level of the individual, researchers can examine within-group as well as between-group differences in the internalization of particular attitudes.

In the end, the models of cultural value orientations and resource exchange presented in this book offer important advantages over alternative models based solely on social group memberships. The linear effects of several cultural values upon patterns of interpersonal resource exchange can be hypothesized, depicted visually, and tested quite readily; in addition, ethnicity can be included as a moderator variable in such models. In contrast, models based solely on social group memberships virtually compel personal relationship researchers to hypothesize complex—and possibly implausible—interaction effects that scarcely can be captured visually and that require sample sizes so large as to make any significant results appear to be trivial from a conceptual standpoint. Part of the appeal of cultural value orientations is that, if ambitious researchers really wanted to test for interaction effects among continuous variables, appropriate methods exist within the LISREL program (Jaccard & Wan, 1996). Thus, the structural equation models of cultural values, ethnicity, and resource exchange presented throughout this book offer a great deal of flexibility to researchers that is not afforded to ANOVA models of social group memberships and resource exchange.

Generalizing the Inclusive Model Across Male-Female Relationships

Aside from the issue of whether cultural value orientations are manifested in personal relationship processes, we may ask whether the "core" model of interpersonal resource exchange presented in Chapter 1 of this volume represents a general relationship process among male-female relationships. If the conceptual core of the inclusive model cannot be supported empirically, then the viability of the entire inclusive model may be called into question. Fortunately, the results of my own studies of interpersonal resource exchange suggest that patterns of resource exchange are characteristic of heterosexual dating and marital relationships, among primarily Anglo samples (Gaines, 1996) and among interethnic samples (Gaines, Rios et al. 1996). Canonical correlation analyses of data from these studies (see Cohen & Cohen, 1983; Harris, 1985; Levine, 1977; Thompson, 1984) lend support to the hypothesis that individuals in romantic relationships reciprocate affectionate and respectful behaviors to a significant degree.

Multivariate tests of significance for canonical correlation analyses of data from the aforementioned study of 112 interethnic heterosexual couples (Gaines, Rios et al., 1996) are presented in Tables 6.1 and 6.2. As Table 6.1 indicates, affection-related behaviors covaried to a significant degree. Similarly as Table 6.2 indicates, respect-related behaviors covaried to a significant degree.

Table 6.1:
Multivariate Tests of Significance for Canonical Correlation Analyses of Men's and Women's Affection-Related Behaviors Among Interethnic Romantic Relationships (*n* = 108 couples)[1]

Test Name	Value	Approx. F	Hypoth. DF	Error DF	p
Pillai's Trace	.58	1.82	36.00	606.00	< .01
Hotelling's T	.78	2.04	36.00	566.00	< .01
Wilk's Lambda	.51	1.94	36.00	424.33	< .01

[1]NOTE: *These analyses were conducted on data collected originally by Gaines, Rios, Granrose, Bledsoe, Farris, Page, and Garcia (1996).*

Table 6.2:
Multivariate Tests of Significance for Canonical Correlation Analyses of Men's and Women's Respect-Related Behaviors Among Interethnic Romantic Relationships (*n* = 111 couples)[2]

Test Name	Value	Approx. F	Hypoth. DF	Error DF	p
Pillai's Trace	.64	2.07	36.00	624.00	< .01
Hotelling's T	.88	2.39	36.00	584.00	< .01
Wilk's Lambda	.47	2.24	36.00	437.50	< .01

[2]NOTE: *These analyses were conducted on data collected originally by Gaines, Rios, Granrose, Bledsoe, Farris, Page, and Garcia (1996).*

Meta-analyses of multivariate tests of significance for the canonical correlation analyses of data from (1) a sample of 62 between-gender friendships (Gaines, 1994), (2) a sample of 219 heterosexual dating relationships (Gaines, 1996), (3) a sample of 106 engaged/married relationships (Gaines, 1996), and (4) a sample of 76 brother-sister relationships (Gaines, Rugg, Zemore, Armm, Yum, Law, Underhill, & Feldman, 1996) are presented in Tables 6.3 and 6.4. (For discussions of meta-analyses, see Rosenthal, 1984; Wolf, 1986.) These samples were grouped together for the purposes of the present chapter, partly because all used a particular set of behavioral items adapted from Foa and Foa (1974) that differed from the items used by Gaines, Rios, Granrose, Bledsoe, Farris, Page, and Garcia (1996), and partly because none of these samples included measures of cultural value orientations (unlike Gaines, Rios et al. 1996). Tables 6.3 and 6.4 indicate that, among all four relationship types, men's and women's respect-related behaviors covaried significantly. In addition, among all relationship types except cross-sex friends, men's and women's affection-related behaviors covaried to a significant degree.

The results of the meta-analyses suggest that exchanges involving respect generalize across romantic cross-sex relationships (both dating and marital) and across nonromantic cross-sex relationships (both family and peer). Also, exchanges involving affection generalize across romantic cross-sex relationships. However, exchanges involving affection appear to be limited to those nonromantic cross-sex relationships that involve family members (rather than peers).

As a whole, personal relationship processes involving interpersonal resource exchange—especially as far as respect is concerned—can be found across a wide variety of male-female relationships. Nevertheless, we cannot say for certain whether such behavioral processes are characteristic of *all* types of male-female relationships. For example, Foa and Foa (1974) hypothesized that mother-son and father-daughter relationships would be characterized by exchanges involving affection but not respect. Such a pattern of reciprocity, if verified empirically, would represent the mirror image of Gaines's (1994a) results for male-female friendships. To date, however, research on interpersonal resource exchange has not focused upon opposite-sex family relationships (except, of course, for husband-wife relationships).

Table 6.3:
Meta-Analytic Summary of Results for Canonical Correlation
Analyses of Men's and Women's Affection-Related Behaviors
Among Cross-Sex Friendships, Dating Relationships, Engaged/
Marital Relationships, and Brother-Sister Relationships[3]

		p		
Test Name	*Sample 1*	*Sample 2*	*Sample 3*	*Sample 4*
Pillai's Trace	.471	.002	.108	.001
Hotelling's T	.364	.001	.084	.000
Wilk's Lambda	.418	.001	.095	.000

		z		
Test Name	*Sample 1*	*Sample 2*	*Sample 3*	*Sample 4*
Pillai's Trace	.05	2.85	1.25	3.00
Hotelling's T	.35	3.00	1.40	4.00
Wilk's Lambda	.20	3.00	1.30	4.00

Test Name	*Overall z*	*Overall p*
Pillai's Trace	3.58	< .01
Hotelling's T	4.38	< .01
Wilk's Lambda	4.25	< .01

[3]NOTE: *Sample 1 = 62 cross-sex friendships (Gaines, 1994).*
Sample 2 = 214 heterosexual dating relationships (Gaines, 1996).
Sample 3 = 106 engaged/marital relationships (Gaines, 1996).
Sample 4 = 76 brother-sister relationships (Gaines, Rugg, Zemore, Armm,
Yum, Law, Underhill, & Feldman, 1996).

Generalizing Beyond Male-Female Relationships

As far as I know, no study has examined cultural value orientations as potential influences on personal relationship processes among romantic or nonromantic same-sex pairs. For instance, virtually nothing is known about patterns of interpersonal resource exchange in gay or lesbian relationships (see Gaines, 1995b; Huston & Schwartz, 1995). My own research on same-sex non-romantic friendships (Gaines, 1994a) indicates that neither affection *nor* respect is reciprocated to a significant degree among male-male or female pairs. Re-

131

Table 6.4:
Meta-Analytic Summary of Results for Canonical Correlation Analyses of Men's and Women's Respect-Related Behaviors Among Cross-Sex Friendships, Dating Relationships, Engaged/ Marital Relationships, and Brother-Sister Relationships[4]

	p			
Test Name	*Sample 1*	*Sample 2*	*Sample 3*	*Sample 4*
Pillai's Trace	.034	.008	.044	.011
Hotelling's T	.025	.005	.034	.002
Wilk's Lambda	.029	.007	.039	.005

	z			
Test Name	*Sample 1*	*Sample 2*	*Sample 3*	*Sample 4*
Pillai's Trace	1.80	2.40	1.70	2.30
Hotelling's T	1.95	2.55	1.80	2.85
Wilk's Lambda	1.90	2.45	1.75	2.55

Test Name	*Overall z*	*Overall p*
Pillai's Trace	4.10	< .01
Hotelling's T	4.58	< .01
Wilk's Lambda	4.33	< .01

[3]NOTE: *Sample 1 = 61 cross-sex friendships (Gaines, 1994).*
Sample 2 = 218 heterosexual dating relationships (Gaines, 1996).
Sample 3 = 106 engaged/marital relationships (Gaines, 1996).
Sample 4 = 76 brother-sister relationships (Gaines, Rugg, Zemore, Armm, Yum, Law, Underhill, & Feldman, 1996).

searchers might find it useful to develop and test hypotheses as to whether patterns of interpersonal resource exchange (or lack thereof) among gay male and/or lesbian relationships resemble those of (1) romantic heterosexual relationships, (2) same-sex friendships, or (3) neither of the above.

We know even less about resource exchange among same-sex family relationships (e.g., father-son, mother-daughter). For example, Foa and Foa (1974) hypothesized that exchanges involving respect, but not affection, would characterize same-sex parent-offspring relationships. However, I do not know of any studies that have tested the Foas's hypotheses in this regard.

Ultimately, research on cultural value orientations and personal relationship processes will need to address the possibility that social exchange theories (including resource exchange theory) and other equity theories fail to account for patterns of interpersonal behavior in romantic *or* nonromantic same-sex relationships. Of course, one could ask whether *any* major social-psychological theories relevant to the study of personal relationships accurately capture the interplay between cultural values and relationship processes. A few studies using the framework of interdependence theory (Kelley & Thibaut, 1978; Thibaut & Kelley, 1959) have addressed issues such as the role of cultural values in moderating the impact of satisfaction, alternatives, and investments on commitment in heterosexual close relationships (Lin & Rusbult, 1995) and the role of cultural values in mediating the impact of ethnicity on responses to co-workers' dissatisfaction regardless of gender (Henderson, 1996). However, neither interdependence theorists nor exchange theorists have examined the full range of cultural values identified in the inclusive model as potential predictors of personal relationship processes in same-sex relationships involving friends or romantic partners.

Final Thoughts

This final section might be appropriately subtitled "Atoms, Automatons, and Matter." In this section, I shall discuss three prevailing themes that implicitly or explicitly have defined the content of this book. Each of these themes, in my opinion, has been neglected within the science of personal relationships.

First, *relationships are not atoms*. As Kenny (1979) observed, the tendency toward reductionism in the natural sciences is counterproductive to the study of personal relationships. By definition, a personal relationship involves two thinking, feeling, acting human beings. Accordingly, all of the models proposed in this book emphasize the dyad, rather than the individual, as the basic unit of analysis. Especially with regard to resource exchange theory, hypotheses should be devised and tested at the level of the dyad (see also Kenny & Kashy, 1991).

Second, *individuals are not automatons.* No conceptual model of personal relationships—including the inclusive model or the more narrowly constructed models presented in this book—is likely to come close to explaining 100% of individual differences in interpersonal behavior (Kenny, 1979; Sobel, 1995). Throughout this book, my collaborators and I have sought to identify person variables (i.e., individuals' internalized cultural value orientations) and situation variables (i.e., partners' interpersonal behavior) as influences on individuals' interpersonal behavior. Nevertheless, we believe that error variance should be acknowledged in any conceptual model of personal relationship processes.

Last but not least, *culture and ethnicity matter.* This third point forms the crux of this book. The possibility that patterns of interpersonal resource exchange and other personal relationship processes are influenced largely by sets of values regarding the welfare of self, community, family, significant others, and living beings as a whole—values that are passed down from generation to generation and that vary in importance partly as a function of ethnicity—deserves more attention within the personal relationship literature than it now draws (Gaines, 1995b). As my colleagues and I have observed elsewhere (e.g., Gaines & Reed, 1994, 1995), if ever we are to transcend ethnicity, we must acknowledge ethnicity in the first place. Only by incorporating a heightened awareness of culture and ethnicity into theories and research will we be able to speak meaningfully about universal models of personal relationship processes.

Contributors

Stanley O. Gaines, Jr., is Assistant Professor in the Department of Psychology, Pomona College, and in the Intercollegiate Department of Black Studies, The Claremont Colleges.

Raymond Buriel is Associate Dean of the College and Professor of Psychology and Chicano Studies at Pomona College.

James H. Liu is lecturer in psychology at Victoria University of Wellington. He received his Ph.D. in social psychology from UCLA in 1992.

Diana I. Ríos is Assistant Professor of Communication and Journalism, The University of New Mexico.

References

Aamott, T. L. & Matthaei, J. A. (1991). *Race, gender and work: A multicultural economic history of women in the United States.* Boston: South End Press.

Abalos, D. T. (1986). *Latinos in the United States: The sacred and the political.* Notre Dame, IN: University of Notre Dame Press.

Acosta, F. X. (1984). Psychotherapy with Mexican Americans: Clinical and empirical gains. In J. L. Martinez, Jr. and R. H. Mendoza (Eds.), *Chicano psychology,* 2nd ed. (Orlando, FL: Academic Press), pp. 163–189.

Acuna, R. (1988). *Occupied America: A history of Chicanos,* 3rd ed. New York: Harper & Row.

Adams, J. S. (1963). Toward an understanding of inequity. *Journal of Abnormal Social Psychology, 67,* 422–436.

Adams, J. S. (1965). Inequity in social exchange. In L. Berkowitz (Ed.), *Advances in experimental social psychology,* vol. 2 (New York: Academic Press), pp. 266–300.

Adams, R. (1937). *Interracial marriage in Hawaii: A study of the mutually conditioned processes of acculturation and amalgamation.* New York: MacMillan.

Adler, A. (1927/1968). *Understanding human nature.* Greenwich, CT: Fawcett.

Agbayani-Siewert, P. & Revilla, L. (1995). Filipino Americans. In P. G. Min (Ed.), *Asian Americans: Contemporary trends and issues* (Thousand Oaks, CA: Sage), pp. 134–168.

Alba, R. D. & Chamlin, M. B. (1983). A preliminary examination of ethnic identification among Whites. *American Sociological Review, 48,* 240–247.

Aldridge, D. P. (1973). The changing nature of interracial marriage in Georgia: A research note. *Journal of Marriage and the Family, 35,* 641–642.

Allman, K. M. (1996). (Un)natural boundaries: Mixed race, gender, and sexuality. In M.P.P. Root (Ed.), *The multiracial experience: Racial borders as the new frontier* (Thousand Oaks, CA: Sage), pp. 277–290.

Allen, E., Jr. (1995). Toward a "more perfect union": A commingling of constitutional ideals and Christian precepts. *The Black Scholar, 25,* 27–34.

Allen, R. L. (1995). Racism, sexism, and a million men. *The Black Scholar, 25,* 24–26.

Allport, G. W. (1954). *The nature of prejudice.* Cambridge, MA: Addison-Wesley.

Aron, A. & Aron, E. N. (1986). *Love and the expansion of self: Understanding attraction and satisfaction.* New York: Hempshire.

Aron, A. & Aron, E. N. (1996). Self and self-expansion in relationships. In G.J.O. Fletcher and J. Fitness (Eds.), *Knowledge structures in close relationships: A social psychological approach* (Mahwah, NJ: Erlbaum), pp. 325–344.

Asante, M. K. (1981). Black male and female relationship: An Afrocentric context. In L. E. Gary (Ed.), *Black men* (Beverly Hills, CA: Sage), pp. 75–82.

Asante, M. K. (1988). *Afrocentricity.* Trenton, NJ: Africa World Press.

Asante, M. K. (1994). The Afrocentric idea. In R. Takaki (Ed.), *From different shores: Perspectives on race and ethnicity in America,* 2nd ed. (New York: Oxford University Press), pp. 283–287.

Atkinson, J. & Huston, T. L. (1984). Sex role orientation and division of labor early in marriage. *Journal of Personality and Social Psychology, 46,* 330–345.

Awkward, M. (1995). *Negotiating difference: Race, gender, and the politics of positionality.* Chicago: University of Chicago Press.

Azibo, D.Y.A. (1989). Pitfalls and some ameliorative strategies in African personality research. *Journal of Black Studies, 19,* 306–319.

Baber, R. (1937). A study of 325 mixed marriages. *American Sociological Review, 2,* 705–716.

Baldwin, J. (1963). *Another country.* New York: Dell.

Ballesteros, D. (1979). Bilingual-bicultural education: A must for Chicanos. In A. D. Trejo (Ed.), *The Chicanos: As we see ourselves* (Tucson: University of Arizona Press), pp. 151–165.

References

Bartz, K. & Levine, E. (1978). Childrearing by Black parents: A description and comparison of Anglo and Chicano parents. *Journal of Marriage and the Family, 40*, 709–719.

Bean, F. D. & Tienda, M. (1987). *The Hispanic population of the United States in the 1980s.* New York: Russell Sage.

Bell, Y. R., Bouie, C. L., & Baldwin, J. A. (1990). Afrocentric cultural consciousness and African-American male-female relationships. *Journal of Black Studies, 21*, 162–189.

Bellah, R. N., Madsen, R., Sullivan, W. M., Swidler, A., & Tipton, S. M. (1985). *Habits of the heart: Individualism and commitment in American life.* Berkeley: University of California Press.

Bem, S. L. (1974). The measurement of psychological androgyny. *Journal of Consulting and Clinical Psychology, 42*, 155–162.

Berscheid, E. (1985). Interpersonal attraction. In G. Lindzey and E. Aronson (Eds.), *The handbook of social psychology*, 3rd ed., vol. 2 (New York: Random House), pp. 413–483.

Berscheid, E. (1994). Interpersonal relationships. *Annual Review of Psychology, 45*, 79–129.

Bianchi, S. M. & Farley, R. (1979). Racial differences in family living arrangements and economic well-being. *Journal of Marriage and the Family, 41*, 537–551.

Billingsley, A. (1968). *Black families in White America.* New York: Simon & Schuster.

Bischof, L. J. (1964). *Interpreting personality theories.* New York: Harper & Row.

Blackwell, J. E. (1985). *The Black community: Diversity and unity*, 2nd ed. New York: Harper & Row.

Blauner, R. (1972). *Racial oppression in America.* New York: Harper & Row.

Blea, I. I. (1988). *Toward a Chicano social science.* New York: Praeger.

Blea, I. I. (1992). *La Chicana and the intersection of race, class, and gender.* New York: Praeger.

Boston, T. D. (1985). *Race, class, and conservatism.* Boston: Unwin Hyman.

Bowman, P. J. (1993). The impact of economic marginality among African American husbands and fathers. In H. P. McAdoo (Ed.), *Family ethnicity: Strength in diversity* (Newbury Park, CA: Sage), pp. 120–137.

Boyd, H. (1995). The march. *The Black Scholar, 25*, 12–16.

Boyd-Franklin, N. & Garcia-Preto, N. (1994). Family therapy: The cases of African American and Hispanic women. In L. Comas-Diaz and B. Greene (Eds.), *Women of color: Integrating ethnic and gender identities in psychotherapy* (New York: Guilford), pp. 239–264.

Bradshaw, C. K. (1994). Asian and Asian American women: Historical and political considerations. In L. Comas-Diaz and B. Greene (Eds.), *Women of color: Integrating ethnic and gender identities in psychotherapy* (New York: Guilford), pp. 72–113.

Braithwaite, V. A. & Scott, W. A. (1991). Values. In J. P. Robinson, P. R. Shaver, and L. S. Wrightsman (Eds.), *Measures of personality and social psychological attitudes* (New York: Academic Press), pp. 661–753.

Brown, R. (1986). *Social psychology*, 2nd ed. New York: Free Press.

Burgess, A. E. (1956). *What price integration?* Dallas: American Guild Press.

Buriel, R. (1984). Integration with traditional Mexican-American culture and sociocultural adjustment. In J. L. Martinez, Jr. and R. H. Mendoza (Eds.), *Chicano psychology*, 2nd ed. (Orlando, FL: Academic Press), pp. 95–130.

Buriel, R. & Cardoza, D. (1988). Sociocultural correlates of achievement among three generations of Mexican American high school seniors. *American Educational Research Journal*, 25, 177–192.

Buriel, R. & Saenz, E. (1980). Psychocultural characteristics of college-bound and noncollege-bound Chicanas. *Journal of Social Psychology*, 110, 245–251.

Burma, J. H. (1952). Research note on the measurement of interracial marriage. *American Journal of Sociology*, 57, 587–589.

Burns, E. B. (1982). *Latin America: A concise interpretive history*, 3rd ed. Englewood Cliffs, NJ: Prentice Hall.

Cabrera, Y. A. (1971). *Emerging faces: The Mexican-Americans*. Dubuque, IA: W. C. Brown.

Carrasco, F. F., Wilkins-Vigil, W. G., & Auslander, N. (1977). *Chicano children and their outdoor environment: Barrio, housing project and rural settings*. Denver: Colorado Program.

Carroll, H. K. (1975). *Report on the island of Porto Rico*. New York: Arno.

Carson, R. C. (1969). *Interaction concepts of personality*. Chicago: Aldine.

Carter, R. T. (1995). *The influence of race and racial identity in psychotherapy: Toward a racially inclusive model*. New York: Wiley-Interscience.

Cha, J. H. (1994). Aspects of individualism and collectivism in Korea. In U. Kim, H. C. Triandis, C. Kagitcibasi, S-C. Choi, and G. Yoon (Eds.), *Individualism and collectivism: Theory, methods, and applications* (Newbury Park, CA: Sage), pp. 157–174.

Champly, H. (1939). *White women, coloured men*. London: J. Long.

Chilman, C. S. (1993). Hispanic families in the United States: Research perspectives. In H. P. McAdoo (Ed.), *Family ethnicity: Strength in diversity* (Newbury Park, CA: Sage), pp. 141–163.

Chimezie, A. (1984). *Black culture: Theory and practice*. Shaker Heights, OH: Keeble Press.

Chin, J. L. (1994). Psychodynamic approaches. In L. Comas-Diaz and B. Greene (Eds.), *Women of color: Integrating ethnic and gender identities in psychotherapy* (New York: Guilford), pp. 194–222.

Chow, E.N.L. (1991). The development of feminist consciousness among Asian American women. In J. Lorber and S. A. Farrell (Eds.), *The social construction of gender* (Newbury Park, CA: Sage), pp. 255–268.

Clark, K. B. (1965). *Dark Ghetto: Dilemmas of social power*. Middletown, CT: Wesleyan University Press.

Clarke, J. J. (1992). *In search of Jung: Historical and philosophical enquiries*. London: Routledge.

Cohen, J. & Cohen, P. (1983). *Applied multiple regression/correlation for the behavioral sciences*. Hillsdale, NJ: Erlbaum.

Collins, R. (1989). Love and property. In J. M. Henslin (Ed.), *Marriage and family in a changing society* (New York: Free Press). pp. 96–104.

Comas-Diaz, L. (1994). An integrative approach. In L. Comas-Diaz and B. Greene (Eds.), *Women of color: Integrating ethnic and gender identities in psychotherapy* (New York: Guilford), pp. 287–318.

Comer-Edwards, A. F. (1988). Mate selection and psychological need. In A. F. Comer-Edwards and J. Spurlock (Eds.), *Black families in crisis: The middle class* (New York: Brunner/Mazel), pp. 37–49.

Cook, N. D. & Kono, S. (1977). Black psychology: The third great tradition. *Journal of Black Psychology*, *3*, 18–28.

Corcoran-Nantes, Y. (1990). Women and popular urban social movements in Sao Pablo, Brazil. *Bulletin of Latin American Research*, *9*, 249–264.

Cortes, C. E. (1986). The education of language minority students: A contextual interaction model. In Bilingual Education Office (California State Department of Education), *Beyond language: Social and cultural factors in schooling language minority students* (Los Angeles: Evaluation, Dissemination, and Assessment Center, California State University), pp. 3–33.

Crohn, J. (1995). *Mixed matches: How to create successful interracial, interethnic, and interfaith relationships*. New York: Fawcett Columbine.

Cromwell, R. E. & Ruiz, R. A. (1979). The myth of macho dominance in decision making within Mexican and Chicano families. *Hispanic Journal of Behavioral Sciences, 1,* 355–373.

Darity, W. A., Jr. & Myers, S. L., Jr. (1984). Does welfare dependency cause female hardship? The case of the Black family. *Journal of Marriage and the Family, 46,* 765–779.

Darwin, L. (1929). *What is eugenics?* New York: Galton.

Davis, S. K. & Chavez, V. (1985). Hispanic househusbands. *Hispanic Journal of Behavioral Sciences, 7,* 317–332.

de Beauvoir, S. (1953). *The second sex.* New York: Knopf.

del Carmen, R. (1990). Assessment of Asian-Americans for family therapy. In F. C. Serafica, A. I. Schwebel, R. K. Russell, P. D. Isaac, and L. B. Myers (Eds.), *Mental health of ethnic minorities* (New York: Praeger), pp. 139–166.

Deutsch, M. & Collins, M. E. (1951). *Interracial housing: A psychological evaluation of a social experiment.* Minneapolis: University of Minnesota Press.

Diaz-Guerrero, R. (1984). The psychological study of the Mexican. In J. L. Martinez, Jr. and R. H. Mendoza (Eds.), *Chicano psychology,* 2nd ed. (Orlando, FL: Academic Press), pp. 95–130.

Dieppa, I. & Montiel, M. (1978). Hispanic families: An introduction. In M. Montiel (Ed.), *Hispanic families: Critical issues for policy and programs in human services* (Washington, DC: National Coalition of Hispanic Mental Health and Human Services Organizations), pp. 1–8.

Dietrich, K. T. (1975). A reexamination of the myth of Black matriarchy. *Journal of Marriage and the Family, 37,* 367–374.

Dion, K. K. & Dion, K. L. (1993). Individualistic and collectivistic perspectives on gender and the cultural context of love and intimacy. *Journal of Social Issues, 49,* 53–69.

Doherty, R. W., Hatfield, E., Thompson, K., & Choo, P. (1994). Cultural and ethnic influences on love and attachment. *Personal Relationships, 1,* 391–398.

Dorman, J. H. (1979). Ethnic groups and "ethnicity": Some theoretical considerations. *Journal of Ethnic Studies, 7,* 23–36.

Du Bois, W.E.B. (1903/1969). *The souls of Black folk.* New York: Signet.

Du Bois, W.E.B. (1921/1975). *Darkwater: Voices from within the veil.* Millwood, NY: Kraus-Thomson.

Du Bois, W.E.B. (1965/1990). *The world and Africa.* New York: International.

Du Bois, W.E.B. (1986). *Writings.* New York: Library of America.

Duck, S. (1986). *Human relationships.* London: Sage.

Duck, S. (1992). *Human relationships,* 2nd ed. London: Sage.

Duck, S. (1994). *Meaningful relationships: Talking, sense, and relating.* Thousand Oaks, CA: Sage.

Durrett, M. E., Richards, P., Otaki, M., Pennebaker, J. W., & Nyquist, L. (1986). Mother's involvement with infant and her perception of spousal support, Japan and America. *Journal of Marriage and the Family, 48,* 187–194.

Edwards, J. N., Fuller, T. D., Sermsri, S., & Vorakitphokatorn, S. (1992). Household crowding and reproductive behavior. *Social Biology, 39,* 212–230.

Ellis, J. A. (1971). *Latin America: Its people and institutions.* New York: Bruce.

Espin, O. M. (1986): Cultural and historical influences on sexuality in Hispanic/Latin women. In J. B. Cole (Ed.), *All American women: Lines that divide, ties that bind* (New York: Free Press), pp. 272–284.

Espiritu, Y. L. (1992). *Asian American panethnicity: Bridging institutions and identities.* Philadelphia: Temple University Press.

Espiritu, Y. L. (1997). *Asian American women and men: Labor, laws, and love.* Thousand Oaks, CA: Sage.

Ewen, R. B. (1993). *An introduction to theories of personality,* 4th ed. Hillsdale, NJ: Erlbaum.

Feagin, J. R. (1991). The continuing significance of race: Antiblack discrimination in public places. *American Sociological Review, 56,* 101–116.

Fehr, B. (1993). How do I love thee? Let me consult my prototype. In S. Duck (Ed.), *Individuals in relationships* (Newbury Park, CA: Sage), pp. 87–120.

Fehr, B. (1994). Prototype-based assessment of laypeople's everyday views of love. *Personal Relationships, 1,* 309–331.

Figueroa-Torres, J. & Pearson, R. E. (1979). Effects of structured learning therapy upon self-control of Puerto Rican fathers. *Hispanic Journal of Behavioral Sciences, 1,* 345–354.

Fischer, A., Beasley, J. D., & Harter, C. L. (1968). The occurrence of the extended family at the origin of the family to procreation: A developmental approach to Negro family structure. *Journal of Marriage and the Family, 30,* 290–300.

Fisher, I., ed. (1980). *The third woman: Minority women writers of the United States.* Boston: Houghton Mifflin.

Flores, J. (1985). "Que assimilated, brother, yo soy asimilao": The structuring of Puerto Rican identity in the U.S. *Journal of Ethnic Studies, 13,* 1–16.

Foa, U. G. & Foa, E. B. (1974). *Societal structures of the mind.* Springfield, IL: Charles C. Thomas.

Frazier, E. F. (1939). *The Negro family in the United States.* Chicago: University of Chicago Press.

Frazier, E. F. (1957). *Black bourgeoisie.* New York: Free Press.

French, M. (1977). *The women's room.* New York: Jove.

French, M. (1985). *Beyond power: On women, men, and morals.* New York: Ballantine.

Freud, S. (1918/1946). *Totem and taboo.* New York: Vintage.

Gaines, S. O., Jr. (1993). *Familism and interpersonal resource exchange among Latinas and Latinos.* Paper presented at the 1993 conference of the National Association for Ethnic Studies, University of Utah, Salt Lake City, March 4–7.

Gaines, S. O., Jr. (1994a). Exchange of respect-denying behaviors among male-female friendships. *Journal of Social and Personal Relationships, 11,* 5–24.

Gaines, S. O., Jr. (1994b). *"Feminism" and interpersonal resource exchange among interethnic couples.* Paper presented at the 1994 conference of the National Association for Ethnic Studies, Kansas City, Missouri, March 16–20.

Gaines, S. O., Jr. (1994c). Generic, stereotypic, and collectivistic models of interpersonal resource exchange among African American couples. *Journal of Black Psychology, 20,* 291–301.

Gaines, S. O., Jr. (1995a). Classifying dating couples: Gender as reflected in traits, roles, and resulting behavior. *Basic and Applied Social Psychology, 16,* 75–94.

Gaines, S. O., Jr. (1995b). Relationships between members of cultural minorities. In J. T. Wood and S. Duck (Eds.), *Under-studied relationships: Off the beaten track* (Thousand Oaks, CA: Sage), pp. 51–88.

Gaines, S. O., Jr. (1996a). Impact of interpersonal traits and gender-role compliance on interpersonal resource exchange among dating and engaged/married couples. *Journal of Social and Personal Relationships, 12,* 241–261.

Gaines, S. O., Jr. (1996b). Perspectives of Du Bois and Fanon on the psychology of oppression. In L. R. Gordon, R. T. White, and T. D. Sharpley-Whiting (Eds.), *Fanon: A critical reader* (Oxford, UK: Basil Blackwell), pp. 24–33.

Gaines, S. O., Jr. (1997). Communalism and the reciprocity of affection and respect among interethnic married couples. *Journal of Black Studies.*

Gaines, S. O., Jr. & Ickes, W. (1996). Perspectives on interracial relationships. In S. Duck (Ed.), *Handbook of personal relationships* (Sussex, UK: Wiley).

Gaines, S. O., Jr. & Jones-Mitchell, J. (1996). Lots of good Black men out there. In N. Ba'Nikongo (Ed.), *Contending issues in African American studies* (Washington, DC: Howard University Press, in press.

Gaines, S. O., Jr., Marelich, W. D., Bledsoe, K. L., Steers, W. N., Henderson, M. C., Granrose, C. S., Barajas, L., Hicks, D., Lyde, M., Takahashi, Y., Yum, N., Rios, D. I., Garcia, B. F.,

Farris, K., Page, M. S. (in press). Racial/Ethnic group differences in cultural value orientations as mediated by racial/ethnic identity and moderated by gender. *Journal of Personality and Social Psychology.*

Gaines, S. O., Jr. & Reed, E. S. (1994). Two social psychologies of prejudice: Gordon W. Allport, W.E.B. Du Bois, and the legacy of Booker T. Washington. *Journal of Black Psychology, 20,* 8–28.

Gaines, S. O., Jr. & Reed, E. S. (1995). Prejudice: From Allport to Du Bois. *American Psychologist, 50,* 96–103.

Gaines, S. O., Jr., Rios, D. I., Granrose, C., Bledsoe, K., Farris, K., Page, M. S., & Garcia, B. (1996). *Romanticism and resource exchange among interethnic/interracial couples.* Paper presented at the 1996 conference of the Social Psychologists in Texas, The University of Texas at Arlington, Jan. 11–12.

Gaines, S. O., Jr., Roberts, D. C., & Baumann, D. J. (1993). When all the world's a stage: The impact of events on news coverage of South Africa, 1979–1985. *Explorations in Ethnic Studies, 16,* 63–74.

Gaines, S. O., Jr., Rugg, M. A., Zemore, S. E., Armm, J. L., Yum, N., Law, A., Underhill, J. M., & Feldman, K. (1996). *Positive instrumentality, positive expressivity, and gender-role compliance as predictors of interpersonal resource exchange among brother-sister pairs.* Paper presented at the 1996 conference of the International Society for the Study of Personal Relationships, Banff, Canada, August 4–8.

Gallagher, B. J., III. (1995). *The sociology of mental illness,* 4th ed. (Englewood Cliffs, NJ: Erlbaum).

Gandara, P. (1982). Passing through the eye of the needle: High-achieving Chicanas. *Hispanic Journal of Behavioral Sciences, 4,* 167–179.

Gary, L. E. (1981). Conclusion. In L. E. Gary (Ed.), *Black men* (Beverly Hills, CA: Sage), pp. 277–292.

Garza, R. T. & Lipton, J. P. (1984). Foundations for a Chicano social psychology. In J. L. Martinez, Jr. and R. H. Mendoza (Eds.), *Chicano psychology,* 2nd ed. (Orlando, FL: Academic Press), pp. 335–365.

Gaudin, J. M., Jr. & Davis, K. B. (1985). Social networks of Black and White rural families: A research report. *Journal of Marriage and the Family, 47,* 1015–1021.

Gelfand, M. J., Triandis, H. C., & Chan, D. K. (1996). Individualism versus collectivism or versus authoritarianism? *European Journal of Social Psychology, 26,* 397–410.

Gernard, R. (1988). *The Cuban Americans.* New York: Chelsea.

Geschwender, J. A. & Carroll-Seguin, R. (1990). Exploding the myth of African-American progress. In M. R. Malson, E. Mudimbe-Boyi, J. F. O'Barr, & M. Wyer (Eds.), *Black women in America: Social science perspectives* (Chicago: University of Chicago Press), pp. 245–263.

Gibbs, J. T. (1988). Young Black males in America: Endangered, embittered, and embattled. In J. T. Gibbs (Ed.), *Young, Black, and male in America: An endangered species* (Dover, MA: Auburn House), pp. 1–36.

Gilgen, A. R. & Cho, J. H. (1979). Performance of Eastern- and Western-oriented college students on the Value Survey and Ways of Life Scale. *Psychological Reports, 45*, 263–268.

Glick, P. C. (1988). Demographic pictures of Black families. In H. P. McAdoo (Ed.), *Black families*, 2nd ed. (Newbury Park, CA: Sage), pp. 111–132.

Goffman, E. (1963). *Stigma: Notes on the management of spoiled identity*. Englewood Cliffs, NJ: Prentice Hall.

Gold, S. J. (1993). Migration and family adjustment: Continuity and change among Vietnamese in the United States. In H. P. McAdoo (Ed.), *Family ethnicity: Strength in diversity* (Newbury Park, CA: Sage), pp. 300–314.

Golden, J. (1954). Patterns of Negro-White intermarriage. *American Sociological Review, 19*, 144–147.

Goldman, M. (1993). The perils of single life in contemporary Japan. *Journal of Marriage and the Family, 55*, 191–204.

Goldwert, M. (1980). *History as neurosis: Paternalism and machismo in Spanish America*. Lahnam, MD: University Press of America.

Goldwert, M. (1982). *Psychic conflict in Spanish America: Six essays on the psychohistory of the region*. Washington, DC: University Press of America.

Gonzales, S. A. (1979). The Chicana perspective: A design for self-awareness. In A. D. Trejo (Ed.), *The Chicanos: As we see ourselves* (Tucson: University of Arizona Press), pp. 81–99.

Gonzales, S. A. (1986). La Chicana: Guadalupe or Malinche. In B. Lindsay (Ed.), *Comparative perspectives of Third World women: The impact of race, sex, and class* (New York: Praeger), pp. 229–250.

Gonzalez, J. T. (1988). Dilemmas of the high-achieving Chicana: The double-bind factor in male/female relationships. *Sex Roles, 18*, 367–380.

Goode, W. J. (1959). The theoretical importance of love. *American Sociological Review, 24*, 38–47.

Gordon, A. I. (1964). *Intermarriage*. Boston: Beacon.

Gray-Little, B. (1982). Marital quality and power processes among Black couples. *Journal of Marriage and the Family, 44*, 633–645.

Guerrero, E. (1993). *Framing Blackness: The African American image in film*. Philadelphia: Temple University Press.

Guthrie, G. M. & Lonner, W. J. (1986). Assessment of personality and psychopathology. In W. J. Lonner and J. W. Berry (Eds.), *Field methods in cross-cultural research* (Beverly Hills, CA: Sage), pp. 231–264.

Gutman, H. G. (1976). *The Black family in slavery and freedom, 1750–1925*. New York: Pantheon.

Haley, A. (1976). *Roots*. Garden City, NY: Doubleday.

Hall, C. S. & Lindzey, C. (1970). *Theories of personality*, 2nd ed. New York: John Wiley.

Hall, L. K. (1981). Support systems and coping patterns. In L. E. Gary (Ed.), *Black men* (Beverly Hills, CA: Sage), pp. 159–167.

Haller, M. H. (1963). *Eugenics: Hereditarian attitudes in American thought*. New Brunswick, NJ: Rutgers University Press.

Hannerz, U. (1977). Growing up male. In D. Y. Wilkinson and R. L. Taylor (Eds.), *The Black male in America: Perspectives on his status in contemporary society* (Chicago: Nelson-Hall), pp. 33–59.

Harris, R. J. (1985). *A primer of multivariate statistics*, 2nd ed. New York: Academic Press.

Harrison, A. O., Wilson, M. N., Pine, C. J., Chan, S. Q., & Buriel, R. (1995). Family ecologies of ethnic minority children. In N. R. Goldberger and J. B. Veroff (Eds.), *The culture and psychology reader* (New York: New York University Press), pp. 292–320.

Hartzer, K. & Franco, J. N. (1985). Ethnicity, division of household tasks and equity in marital roles: A comparison of Anglo and Mexican American couples. *Hispanic Journal of Behavioral Sciences, 7*, 333–344.

Harvey, J. H., Hendrick, S. S., & Tucker, K. (1988). Self-report methods in studying personal relationships. In S. W. Duck (Ed.), *Handbook of personal relationships* (Chichester, UK: Wiley), pp. 99–113.

Hawkes, G. F. & Taylor, M. (1975). Power structure in Mexican and Mexican-American farm labor families. *Journal of Marriage and the Family, 37*, 807–811.

Hayner, N. S. (1954). The family in Mexico. *Marriage and Family Living, 16*, 369–373.

Heer, D. M. (1974). The prevalence of Black-White marriage in the United States. *Journal of Marriage and the Family, 36*, 246–258.

Heider, F. (1958). *The psychology of interpersonal relations*. Hillsdale, NJ: Erlbaum.

Helms, J. E. (1990). Three perspectives on counseling and psychotherapy with visible racial/ethnic group clients. In F. C. Ser-

References

afica, A. I. Schwebel, R. K. Russell, P. D. Isaac, and L. B. Myers (Eds.), *Mental health of ethnic minorities* (New York: Praeger), pp. 171–201.

Henderson, M. C. (1996). *The impact of ethnicity and cultural value orientations on responses to conflict with co-workers.* Unpublished masters thesis, The Claremont Graduate School, Claremont, CA, May 1996.

Hernton, C. C. (1965). *Sex and racism in America.* Garden City, NY: Doubleday.

Herskovits, M. J. (1935). Social history of the Negro. In C. Murchison (Ed.), *A handbook of social psychology,* Vol. 1 (New York: Russell & Russell), pp. 207–267.

Hill, M. C. (1957). Research on the Negro family. *Marriage and Family Living, 19,* 25–31.

Hill, R. B., with Billingsley, A., Engram., E., Malson, M. R., Rubin, R. H., Stack, C. B., Stewart, J. B., & Teele, J. E. (1993). *Research on the African-American family: A holistic perspective.* Westport, CT: Auburn House.

Hoffereth, S. L. (1984). Kin networks, race, and family structure. *Journal of Marriage and the Family, 46,* 791–806.

Homans, G. C. (1961). *Social behavior: Its elementary forms.* New York: Harcourt Brace.

hooks, b. (1981). *Ain't I a woman: Black women and feminism.* Boston: South End Press.

hooks, b. (1992). *Black looks: Race and representation.* Boston: South End Press.

Hopson, D. S. & Hopson, D. P. (1995). *Friends, lovers, and soul mates: A guide to better relationships between Black men and women.* New York: Fireside.

Horney, K. (1967). *Feminine psychology.* New York: Norton.

Howitt, D. & Owusu-Bempah, J. (1994). *The racism of psychology.* New York: Harvester/Wheatsheaf.

Hur, K. K. & Proudlove, S. J. (1982). *The media behavior of Asian Americans.* Paper presented at the annual convention of the Association for Education in Journalism, Athens, Ohio, July.

Hurtado, A., Rodriguez, J., Gurin, P., & Beals, J. L. (1993). The impact of Mexican descendants' social identity on the ethnic socialization of children. In M. E. Bernal and G. P. Knight (Eds.), *Ethnic identity: Formation and transmission among Hispanics and other minorities* (Albany: State University of New York Press), pp. 131–162.

Huston, M. & Schwartz, P. (1995). The relationships of lesbians and gay men. In J. T. Wood and S. Duck (Eds.), *Under-studied relationships: Off the beaten track* (Thousand Oaks, CA: Sage), pp. 89–121.

Huston, T. L. & Geis, G. (1993). In what ways do gender-related attributes and beliefs affect marriage? *Journal of Social Issues, 49,* 87–106.

Ickes, W. (1984). Compositions in Black and White: Determinants of interaction in interracial dyads. *Journal of Personality and Social Psychology, 47,* 330–341.

Ickes, W. (1985). Sex-role influences on compatibility in relationships. In W. Ickes (Ed.), *Compatible and incompatible relationships* (New York: Springer-Verlag), pp. 187–208.

Ickes, W. (1993). Traditional gender roles: Do they make, and then break, our relationships? *Journal of Social Issues, 49,* 71–85.

Iwao, S. (1993). *The Japanese woman: Traditional image and changing reality.* New York: Macmillan.

Jaccard, J. & Wan, C. K. (1996). *LISREL approaches to interaction effects in multiple regression.* Thousand Oaks, CA: Sage.

Jackson, A. M. (1983). A theoretical model for the practice of psychotherapy with Black populations. *Journal of Black Psychology, 10,* 19–27.

Jacobson, N. S. & Margolin, G. (1979). *Marital therapy: Strategies based on social learning and behavior exchange principles.* New York: Brunner/Mazel.

Jenkins, A. H. (1995). *Psychology and African Americans: A humanistic approach,* 2nd ed. Boston: Allyn and Bacon.

Johnson, L. B. (1988). Perspectives on Black family empirical research: 1965–1978. In H. P. McAdoo (Ed.), *Black families,* 2nd ed. (Newbury Park, CA: Sage), pp. 91–106.

Johnson, M. P., Huston, T. L., Gaines, S. O., Jr., & Levinger, G. (1992). Patterns of married life among young couples. *Journal of Social and Personal Relationships, 9,* 343–364.

Johnson, R. C. & Nagoshi, C. T. (1986). The adjustment of offspring of within-group and interracial/intercultural marriages: A comparison of personality factor scores. *Journal of Marriage and the Family, 48,* 279–284.

Johnston, J. H. (1939). *Miscegenation in the ante-bellum South.* Chicago: University of Chicago Press.

Jones, J. M. (1987). Racism in Black and White: A bicultural model of reaction and evolution. In P. A. Katz and D. A. Taylor (Eds.), *Eliminating racism: Profiles in controversy* (New York: Plenum Press), pp. 117–135.

Joreskog, K. G. & Sorbom, D. (1979). *Advances in factor analysis and structural equation models.* Cambridge, MA: Abt Books.

Joreskog, K. G. & Sorbom, D. (1989). *LISREL 7: A guide to the program and applications,* 2nd ed. Chicago: SPSS Inc.

Jung, C. G. (1978). *Psychology and the East.* Princeton, NJ: Princeton University Press.

Kami, C. K. & Radin, N. L. (1967). Class differences in the social-ization practices of Negro mothers. *Journal of Marriage and the Family, 29,* 302–310.

Kamo, Y. (1993). Determinants of marital satisfaction: A compari-son of the United States and Japan. *Journal of Social and Per-sonal Relationships, 10,* 551–568.

Karenga, M. (1995). The Million Man March/Day of Absence mis-sion statement. *The Black Scholar, 25,* 2–11.

Kelley, H. H. & Thibaut, J. W. (1978). *Interpersonal relations: A theory of interdependence.* New York: Wiley-Interscience.

Kenny, D. A. (1979). *Correlation and causality.* New York: Wiley-Interscience.

Kenny, D. A. (1988). The analysis of data from two-person rela-tionships. In S. W. Duck (Ed.), *Handbook of personal relation-ships* (Chichester, UK: Wiley), pp. 57–77.

Kenny, D. A. & Kashy, D. A. (1991). Analyzing interdependence in dyads. In B. M. Montgomery and S. Duck (Eds.), *Studying in-terpersonal interaction* (New York: Guilford), pp. 275–285.

Kephart, W. M. & Jedlicka, W. M. (1988). *The family, society, and the individual,* 6th ed. New York: Harper & Row.

Kibria, N. (1993). *Family tightrope: The changing lives of Viet-namese Americans.* Princeton, NJ: Princeton University Press.

Kim, E. H. (1986). With silk wings: Asian American women at work. In J. B. Cole (Ed.), *All American women: Lines that di-vide, ties that bind* (New York: Free Press), pp. 95–100.

Kimmel, D. C. (1974). *Adulthood and aging: An interdisciplinary view.* New York: Wiley.

King, K. (1969). Adolescent perception of power structure in the Ne-gro family. *Journal of Marriage and the Family, 31,* 751–755.

Kiram, E. G., Green, V., & Valencia-Weber, G. (1982). Accultura-tion and the Hispanic woman: Attitudes toward women, sex-role attribution, sex-role behavior, and demographics. *Hispanic Journal of Behavioral Sciences, 4,* 21–40.

Kitano, H. H. L. & Daniels, R. (1988). *Asian Americans: Emerging minorities.* Englewood Cliffs, NJ: Prentice Hall.

Kitano, H. H. L., Yeung, W., Chai, L., & Hatanaka, H. (1984). Asian-American interracial marriage. *Journal of Marriage and the Family, 46,* 179–190.

Kluckhohn, F. R. & Strodtbeck, F. L. (1961). *Variations in value ori-entations.* Evanston, IL: Peterson.

Knight, T. J. (1979). *Latin America comes of age.* Metuchen, NJ: Scarecrow Press.

Kriesberg, L. (1967). Rearing children for educational achievement in fatherless homes. *Journal of Marriage and the Family, 29,* 288–301.

L'Abate, L. & Harel, T. (1991). Deriving, developing, and expanding a theory of developmental competence from resource exchange theory. In U. G. Foa, J. Converse, Jr., K. Y. Tornblom, and E. B. Foa (Eds.), *Resource theory: Explorations and applications* (San Diego, CA: Academic Press), pp. 233–269.

Labov, T. & Jacobs, J. A. (1986). Intermarriage in Hawaii. *Journal of Marriage and the Family, 48,* 79–88.

Lammermeier, P. J. (1973). The urban Black family of the nineteenth century: A study of Black family structure in the Ohio Valley. *Journal of Marriage and the Family, 35,* 51–57.

Landrine, H. & Klonoff, E. A. (1996). *African American acculturation: Deconstructing race and reviving culture.* Thousand Oaks, CA: Sage.

Lara-Cantu, M. A. (1989). A sex role inventory with scales for "machismo" and "self-sacrificing woman." *Journal of Cross-Cultural Psychology, 20,* 386–398.

Lara-Cantu, M. A. & Navarro-Arias, R. (1986). Positive and negative factors in the measurement of sex roles: Findings from a Mexican sample. *Hispanic Journal of Behavioral Sciences, 8,* 143–155.

Lebra, T. S. (1994). Mother and child in Japanese socialization: A Japan-U.S. comparison. In P. A. Greenfield and R. Cocking (Eds.), *Cross-cultural roots of minority child development* (Hillsdale, NJ: Erlbaum), pp. 259–274.

Lee, J. A. (1976). *The colors of love.* New York: Prentice Hall.

Lee, J.F.J. (1991). *Asian American experiences in the United States.* Jefferson, NC: McFarland.

Lemelle, S. J. (1993). The politics of cultural existence: Pan-Africanism, historical materialism, and Afrocentricity. *Race and Class, 35,* 93–112.

Levine, E. S. & Bartz, K. W. (1979). Comparative child-rearing attitudes among Chicano, Anglo, and Black parents. *Hispanic Journal of Behavioral Sciences, 1,* 165–178.

Levine, M. S. (1977). *Canonical analysis and factor comparison.* Newbury Park, CA: Sage.

Lewin, K. (1936). *Principles of topographical psychology.* New York: McGraw-Hill.

Lewis, G. K. (1963). *Puerto Rico: Freedom and power in the Caribbean.* New York: Harper Torch Books.

Lewis, O. (1959). *Five families: Mexican case studies in the culture of poverty.* New York: Basic Books.

Lewis, O. (1963). *La vida: A Puerto Rican family in the culture of poverty—San Juan and New York.* New York: Random House.

Liebman, S. B. (1976). *Exploring the Latin American mind.* Chicago: Nelson-Hall.

References

Lin, C. & Liu, W. T. (1993). Intergenerational relationships among Chinese immigrant families from Taiwan. In H. P. McAdoo (Ed.), *Family ethnicity: Strength in diversity* (Thousand Oaks, CA: Sage), pp. 271–286.

Lin, Y. W. & Rusbult, C. E. (1995). Commitment to dating relationships and cross-sex friendships in America and China. *Journal of Social and Personal Relationships, 12,* 7–26.

Loehlin, J. C. (1992). *Latent variable models,* 2nd ed. Hillsdale, NJ: Erlbaum.

Long, J. S. (1983a). *Confirmatory factor analysis: A preface to LIS-REL.* Beverly Hills, CA: Sage.

Long, J. S. (1983b). *Covariance structure analysis: An introduction to LISREL.* Beverly Hills, CA: Sage.

Lucero-Trujillo, M. C. (1980). The dilemma of the modern Chicana artist and critic. In D. Fisher (Ed.), *The third woman: Minority women writers of the United States* (Dallas: Houghton Mifflin), pp. 324–331.

Lyman, S. M. (1994). *Color, culture, civilization: Race and minority issues in American society.* Urbana: University of Illinois Press.

Malveaux, J. (1988). The economic statuses of Black families. In H. P. McAdoo (ED.), *Black families,* 2nd ed. (Newbury Park, CA: Sage), pp. 133–147.

Marable, M. (1986). *W. E. B. Du Bois: Black radical Democrat.* Boston: Twayne.

Marable, M. (1992). *The crisis of color and democracy.* Monroe, ME: Common Courage Press.

Marchetti, G. (1993). *Romance and the "yellow peril": Race, sex, and discursive strategies in Hollywood fiction.* Berkeley: University of California Press.

Margolis, M. L. (1984). *Mothers and such: Views of American women and why they changed.* Berkeley: University of California Press.

Marin, G. (1993). Influences of acculturation on familialism and self-identification among Hispanics. In M. E. Bernal and G. P. Knight (Eds.), Ethnic identity: Formation and transmission among Hispanics and other minorities (Albany: State University of New York Press), pp. 181–196.

Marin, G. & Marin, B. V. (1991). *Research with Hispanic populations.* Newbury Park, CA: Sage.

Marmour, J. (1951). Psychological trends in American family relationships. *Marriage and Family Living, 13,* 145–147.

Martin, E. P. & Martin, J. M. (1978). *The Black extended family.* Chicago: University of Chicago Press.

Matsui, Y. (1989). *Women's Asia.* London: Zed Books.

Mayo, S. H. (1978). *A history of Mexico from pre-Columbia to present.* Englewood Cliffs, NJ: Prentice Hall.

McAdoo, H. P. (1978). Factors related to stability in upwardly mobile Black families. *Journal of Marriage and the Family, 40*, 761–776.

McAdoo, H. P. (1986). Societal stress: The Black family. In J. B. Cole (Ed.), *All American women: Lines that divide, ties that bind* (New York: Free Press), pp. 187–197.

McAdoo, H. P. (1993). Ethnic families: Strengths that are found in diversity. In H. P. McAdoo (Ed.), *Family ethnicity: Strength in diversity* (Newbury Park, CA: Sage), pp. 3–14.

McAdoo, J. L. (1993). Decision making and marital satisfaction in African American families. In H. P. McAdoo (Ed.), *Family ethnicity: Strength in diversity* (Newbury Park, CA: Sage), pp. 109–119.

McCall, G. J. & Simmons, J. L. (1991). Levels of analysis: The individual, the dyad, and the larger social group. In B. M. Montgomery and S. Duck (Eds.), *Studying interpersonal interaction* (New York: Guilford), pp. 56–81.

McClelland, D. C. (1987). *Human motivation.* Cambridge, UK: Cambridge University Press.

McGinn, N. F. (1966). Marriage and female in middle-class Mexico. *Journal of Marriage and the Family, 28*, 305–313.

Meier, M. S. & Ribera, F. (1993). *Mexican Americans, American Mexicans: From conquistadores to Chicanos.* New York: Hill and Wang.

Melton, W. & Thomas, D. L. (1976). Instrumental and expressive values in mate selection of Black and White college students. *Journal of Marriage and the Family, 38*, 509–517.

Menchaca, M. (1989). Chicano-Mexican cultural assimilation and Anglo-Saxon cultural dominance. *Hispanic Journal of Behavioral Sciences, 11*, 203–231.

Milliones, J. (1980). Construction of a Black consciousness measure: Psychotherapeutic implications. *Psychotherapy: Theory, Research, and Practice, 17*, 175–182.

Min, P. G. (1993). Korean immigrants' marital patterns and marital adjustments. In H. P. McAdoo (Ed.), *Family ethnicity: Strength in diversity* (Newbury Park, CA: Sage), pp. 287–299.

Min, P. G. (1995a). An overview of Asian Americans. In P. G. Min (Ed.), *Asian Americans: Contemporary trends and issues* (Thousand Oaks, CA: Sage), pp. 10–37.

Min, P. G. (1995b). Korean Americans. In P. G. Min (Ed.), *Asian Americans: Contemporary trends and issues* (Thousand Oaks, CA: Sage), pp. 199–231.

Mindel, C. H. (1980). Extended familism among urban Mexican Americans, Anglos, and Blacks. *Hispanic Journal of Behavioral Sciences, 2*, 21–34.

References

Miranda, M. R. (1984). Mental health and the Chicano elderly. In J. L. Martinez, Jr. and R. H. Mendoza (Eds.), *Chicano psychology*, 2nd ed. (Orlando, FL: Academic Press), pp. 207–221.

Mirande, A. (1977). The Chicano family: A reanalysis of conflicting values. *Journal of Marriage and the Family, 39*, 747–756.

Mirande, A. (1985). *The Chicano experience: An alternative perspective*. Notre Dame, IN: University of Notre Dame Press.

Mirande, A. & Enriquez, E. (1979). *La Chicana: The Mexican-American woman*. Chicago: University of Chicago Press.

Miyuki, M. (1985a). A reflection on my thirtieth year in the West. In M. Spiegelman and M. Miyuki (Eds.), *Buddhism and Jungian psychology* (Phoenix, AZ: Falcon Press), pp. 15–25.

Miyuki, M. (1985b). The psychodynamics of Buddhist meditation: A Jungian perspective. In M. Spiegelman and M. Miyuki (Eds.), *Buddhism and Jungian psychology* (Phoenix, AZ: Falcon Press), pp. 157–184.

Moacanin, R. C. (1986). *Jung's psychology and Tibetan Buddhism: Western and Eastern paths to the heart*. London: Wisdom Books.

Moghaddan, F. M. (1987). Psychology in the Three Worlds as reflected in the crisis in social psychology and the move toward indigenous Third-World psychology. *American Psychologist, 42*, 912–920.

Moore, J. W. & Pachon, H. (1985). *Hispanics in the United States*. Englewood Cliffs, NJ: Prentice Hall.

Morton, P. (1991). *Disfigured images: The historical assault on Afro-American women*. New York: Praeger.

Myers, L. J. (1985). Transpersonal psychology: The role of the Afrocentric paradigm. *Journal of Black Psychology, 12*, 31–42.

Myers, L. J. (1993). *Understanding an Afrocentric world view: Introduction to an optimal psychology*. Dubuque, IA: Kendall/Hunt.

National Research Council (1989). *A common destiny: Blacks and American society*. Washington, DC: National Academy Press.

Newcomb, T. M. (1956). The prediction of interpersonal attraction. *American Psychologist, 11*, 577–586.

Nobles, W. W. (1978). Toward an empirical and theoretical framework for defining Black families. *Journal of Marriage and the Family, 40*, 679–688.

Nobles, W. W. (1986). *African psychology: Toward its reclamation, reascension, and revitalization*. Oakland, CA: Black Family Institute.

Nye, R. D. (1986). *Three psychologies: Perspectives from Freud, Skinner, and Rogers*, 3rd ed. Monterey, CA: Brooks/Cole.

O'Brien, D. J. & Fugita, S. S. (1991). *The Japanese American experience*. Bloomington: Indiana University Press.

154

Okihiro, G. Y. (1994). *Margins and mainstreams: Asians in American society*. Seattle, WA: University of Washington Press.

Osborn, H. F. (1923). Address of welcome. In Second International Congress of *Eugenics, Eugenics, genetics, and the family* (Baltimore: Williams & Wilkins), pp. 1–4.

Ou, Y. & McAdoo, H. P. (1993). Socialization of Chinese American children. In H. P. McAdoo (Ed.), *Family ethnicity: Strength in diversity* (Thousand Oaks, CA: Sage), pp. 245–270.

Paloutzian, R. F. & Kirkpatrick, L. A. (1995). Introduction: The scope of religious influences on personal and societal well-being. *Journal of Social Issues, 51*, 1–11.

Paredes, A. (1993). *Folklore and culture on the Texas-Mexican border*. Austin, TX: Center for Mexican American Studies, University of Texas at Austin.

Parham, T. A. (1993). *Psychological storms: The African American struggle for identity*. Chicago: African American Images.

Parham, T. A. & Helms, J. E. (1981). The influence of Black students' racial identity on preferences for counselor's race. *Journal of Counseling Psychology, 28*, 250–257.

Parker, S. & Kleiner, R. J. (1966). Characteristics of Negro mothers in single-headed households. *Journal of Marriage and the Family, 28*, 507–513.

Pavela, T. H. (1964). An exploratory study of Negro-White intermarriage in Indiana. *Journal of Marriage and the Family, 26*, 209–211.

Paz, J. J. (1993). Support of Hispanic elderly. In H. P. McAdoo (Ed.), *Family ethnicity: Strength in diversity* (Newbury Park, CA: Sage), pp. 177–183.

Penalosa, F. (1968). Mexican family roles. *Journal of Marriage and the Family, 30*, 680–689.

Pettigrew, T. F. (1964). *A profile of the Negro American*. Princeton, NJ: D. Van Nostrand.

Phinney, J. S. (1996). When we talk about American ethnic groups, what do we mean? *American Psychologist, 51*, 918–927.

Pierson, D. (1954). The family in Brazil. *Marriage and Family Living, 16*, 308–314.

Porterfield, E. (1978). *Black and White mixed marriages*. Chicago: Nelson-Hall.

Powell, L. C. (1983). Black macho and Black feminism. In B. Smith (Ed.), *Home girls: A Black feminist anthology* (New York: Women of Color Press), pp. 283–292.

Puryear, G. R. (1980). The Black woman: Liberated or oppressed: In B. Lindzay (Ed.), *Comparative perspectives of Third World women: The impact of race, sex, and class* (New York: Praeger), pp. 251–275.

References

Radcliffe, S. A. (1990). Multiple identities and negotiation over gender: Female peasant union leaders in Peru. *Bulletin of Latin American Research*, 9, 229–247.

Ramirez, A. (1977). Chicano Power and interracial group relations. In J. L. Martinez, Jr. (Ed.), *Chicano psychology* (New York: Academic Press), pp. 87–96.

Ramirez, M., III. (1983). *Psychology of the Americas: Mestizo perspectives on personality and mental health*. New York: Pergamon Press.

Ramirez, M., III. (1984). Assessing and understanding biculturalism-multiculturalism in Mexican-American adults. In J. L. Martinez, Jr. and R. H. Mendoza (Eds.), *Chicano psychology*, 2nd ed. (Orlando, FL: Academic Press), pp. 77–94.

Ramirez, M., III. (1991). *Psychotherapy and counseling with minorities: A cognitive approach to individual and cultural differences*. New York: Pergamon Press.

Ramos, R. and Ramos, M. (1979). The Mexican American: Am I who they say I am? In A. D. Trejo (Ed.), *The Chicanos: As we see ourselves* (Tucson, AZ: University of Arizona Press), pp. 49–66.

Reed, E. S. (1996). Selves, values, and cultures. In E. S. Reed, E. Turiel, and T. Brown (Eds.), *Values and knowledge* (Hillsdale, NJ: Erlbaum), pp. 1–15.

Reuter, E. B. (1918). *The mulatto in the United States*. Boston: Richard G. Badger.

Rindfuss, R. R., Liao, T. F., & Tsuya, N. O. (1992). Contact with parents in Japan: Effects on opinions toward gender and intergenerational roles. *Journal of Marriage and the Family*, 54, 812–822.

Rios, D. I. (1993). *Mexican American audiences: A qualitative and quantitative study of ethnic subgroup uses for mass media*. Unpublished doctoral dissertation, University of Texas at Austin.

Rios, D. I. (1994). Mexican American cultural experiences with mass mediated communication. In A. Gonzalez, M. Houston, and V. Chen (Eds.), *Voices from within: Explorations in culture, ethnicity, and communication* (Los Angeles: Roxbury), pp. 110–116.

Rodriguez, H. (1992). Household composition, employment patterns, and income inequality: Puerto Ricans in New York and other areas of the U.S. mainland. *Hispanic Journal of Behavioral Sciences*, 14, 52–75.

Rogers, C. R. (1961). *On becoming a person: A therapist's view of psychotherapy*. Boston: Houghton Mifflin.

Rogers, C. R. (1972). *Becoming partners: Marriage and its alternatives*. New York: Delacorte Press.

Rogers, C. R. (1989). *Selections: The Carl Rogers reader*. Boston: Houghton Mifflin.

Roopnairne, J. L., Talukder, E., Jain, D., Joshi, P., & Srivastav, P. (1992). Personal well-being, kinship tie, and mother-infant and father-infant interactions in single-wage and dual-wage families in New Delhi, India. *Journal of Marriage and the Family, 54*, 293–301.

Root, M. P. P. (1992). Within, between, and beyond race. In M. P. P. Root (Ed.), *Racially mixed people in America* (Newbury Park, CA: Sage), pp. 3–11.

Rosenblatt, P. C., Karis, T. A., & Powell, R. D. (1995). *Multiracial couples: Black and White voices*. Thousand Oaks, CA: Sage.

Rosenthal, R. (1984). *Meta-analytic procedures for social research*. Beverly Hills, CA: Sage.

Rueschenberg, E. & Buriel, R. (1989). Mexican American family functioning and acculturation: A family systems perspective. *Hispanic Journal of Behavioral Sciences, 11*, 232–244.

Samoiloff, L. C. (1984). *Portrait of Puerto Rico*. New York: Cornwall.

Sanchez, G. J. (1993). *Becoming Mexican American: Ethnicity, culture, and identity in Chicano Los Angeles, 1900–1945*. New York: Oxford University Press.

Sanchez-Ayendez, M. (1986). Puerto Rican elderly women: Shared meanings and informal supportive networks. In J. B. Cole (Ed.), *All American women: Lines that divide, ties that bind* (New York: Free Press), pp. 172–186.

Sanjek, R. (1994). Intermarriage and the future of races in the United States. In S. Gregory and R. Sanjek (Eds.), *Race* (New Brunswick, NJ: Rutgers University Press), pp. 103–130.

Savage, J. E., Adair, A. V., & Friedman, P. (1978). Community-social variables related to Black parent-abuse homes. *Journal of Marriage and the Family, 40*, 779–785.

Schaefer, R. T. (1988). *Racial and ethnic groups*, 3rd ed. Glenview, IL: Scott, Foresman.

Schellenberg, J. A. (1978). *Masters of social psychology: Freud, Mead, Lewin, and Skinner*. New York: Oxford University Press.

Schmidt, A. & Padilla, A. M. (1983). Grandparent-grandchild interaction in a Mexican-American group. *Hispanic Journal of Behavioral Sciences, 5*, 181–198.

Schoen, R. & Thomas, B. (1989). Intergroup marriage in Hawaii, 1969–1971 and 1979–1981. *Sociological Perspectives, 32*, 365–382.

Schultz, D. A. (1977). Coming up as a boy in the ghetto. In D. Y. Wilkinson and R. L. Taylor (Eds.), *The Black male in America: Perspectives on his status in contemporary society* (Chicago: Nelson-Hall), pp. 7–32.

References

Sellers, R. M. (1993). A call to arms for researchers studying racial identity. *Journal of Black Psychology, 19*, 327–332.

Sena-Rivera, J. (1979). Extended kinship in the United States: Competing models and the case of la familia Chicana. *Journal of Marriage and the Family, 41*, 121–129.

Serafica, F. C. (1990). Counseling Asian-American families: A cultural-developmental approach. In F. C. Serafica, A. I. Schwebel, R. K. Russell, P. D. Isaac, and L. B. Myers (Eds.), *Mental health of ethnic minorities* (New York: Praeger), pp. 222–224.

Shinagawa, L. H. & Pang, G. Y. (1988). Intraethnic, interethnic, and interracial marriages among Asian Americans in California. Berkeley *Journal of Sociology, 33*, 95–114.

Shukla, A. (1987). Decision-making in single- and dual-career families in India. *Journal of Marriage and the Family, 49*, 621–629.

Sjostrom, B. R. (1988). Culture contact and value orientations: The Puerto Rican experience. In E. Acosta-Belin & B. R. Sjostrom (Eds.), *The Hispanic experience in the United States: Contemporary issues and perspectives* (New York: Praeger), pp. 163–186.

Skinner, E. P. (1987). Personal networks and institutional linkages in the global system. In A. M. Cromwell (Ed.), *Dynamics of the African/Afro-American connection* (Washington, DC: Howard University Press), pp. 15–31.

Smith, M. B. (1991). *Values, selves, and society: Toward a humanistic social psychology.* New Brunswick, NJ: Transaction Publishers.

Snyder, M. & Ickes, W. (1985). Personality and social behavior. In G. Lindzey and E. Aronson (Eds.), *The handbook of social psychology*, 3rd ed., vol. 2 (New York: Random House), pp. 883–947.

Sobel, M. E. (1995). Causal inference in the social and behavioral sciences. In G. Arminger, C. C. Clogg, and M. E. Sobel (Eds.), *Handbook of statistical modeling for the social and behavioral sciences* (New York: Plenum Press), pp. 1–38.

Sollors, W. (1986). *Beyond ethnicity: Consent and descent in American culture.* New York: Oxford University Press.

Soto, E. & Shaver, P. (1982). Sex-role traditionalism, assertiveness, and symptoms of Puerto Rican women living in the United States. *Hispanic Journal of Behavioral Sciences, 4*, 1–19.

Spence, J. T., Deaux, K., & Helmreich, R. L. (1985). Sex roles in contemporary American society. In G. Lindzey and E. Aronson (Eds.), *The handbook of social psychology*, 3rd ed., vol. 2 (New York: Random House), pp. 149–178.

Spence, J. T., Helmreich, R. L., & Holahan, C. K. (1979). Negative and positive components of psychological masculinity and femininity and their relationships to self-reports of neurotic and acting-out behaviors. *Journal of Personality and Social Psychology, 37*, 1673–1682.

Spence, J. T., Helmreich, R. L., & Stapp, J. (1974). The Personal Attributes Questionnaire: A measure of sex-role stereotypes and masculinity-femininity. *JSAS Selected Catalog of Documents in Psychology, 4*, 43.

Spickard, P. R. (1989). *Mixed blood: Intermarriage and ethnic identity in twentieth-century America*. Madison: University of Wisconsin Press.

Spigner, C. (1992). *Black female/male relationships, functionalism, and the media*. Paper presented at the 20th Annual Conference of the National Association for Ethnic Studies, Florida Atlantic University, Boca Raton, March 5–8.

Sprecher, S., Aron, A., Hatfield, E., Cortese, A., Potapova, E., Levitskaya, A. (1994). Love: American style, Russian style, and Japanese style. *Personal Relationships, 1*, 349–369.

Stack, S. (1992). The effect of divorce on suicide in Japan: A time series analysis, 1950–1980. *Journal of Marriage and the Family, 54*, 327–334.

Staples, R. (1971). Toward a sociology of the Black family: A theoretical and methodological assessment. *Journal of Marriage and the Family, 33*, 119–138.

Staples, R. (1972). The matricentric family system: A cross-cultural examination. *Journal of Marriage and the Family, 34*, 156–165.

Staples, R. (1977). The myth of the impotent Black male. In D. Y. Wilkinson and R. L. Taylor (Eds.), *The Black male in America: perspectives on his status in contemporary society* (Chicago: Nelson-Hall), pp. 133–144.

Staples, R. (1985). Change in Black family structure: The conflict between family ideology and structural conditions. *Journal of Marriage and the Family, 47*, 1005–1013.

Staples, R. (1994). Interracial relationships: A convergence of desire and opportunity. In R. Staples (Ed.), *The Black family: Essays and studies* (Belmont, CA: Wadsworth), pp. 11–19.

Staples, R. & Mirande, A. (1980). Racial and cultural variations among American families: A decennial review of the literature on minority families. *Journal of Marriage and the Family, 42*, 887–903.

Stember, C. H. (1976). Sexual racism. New York: Harper & Row.

Stephan, C. W. & Stephan, W. G. (1985). *Two social psychologies: An integrative approach*. Homewood, IL: Dorsey Press.

Stephan, C. W. & Stephan, W. G. (1989). After intermarriage: Ethnic identity among mixed-heritage Japanese-Americans and Hispanics. *Journal of Marriage and the Family, 51*, 507–519.

Stephan, W. G. (1985). Intergroup relations. In G. Lindzey and E. Aronson (Eds.), *The handbook of social psychology*, 3rd ed., vol. 2 (New York: Random House), pp. 599–658.

Stevens, E. P. (1973). The prospects for a women's liberation movement in Latin America. *Journal of Marriage and the Family, 35,* 313–330.

Suarez, Z. E. (1993). Cuban Americans: From golden exiles to social undesirables. In H. P. McAdoo (Ed.), *Family ethnicity: Strength in diversity* (Newbury Park, CA: Sage), pp. 164–176.

Sudarkasa, N. (1993). Female-headed African American households: Some neglected dimensions. In H. P. McAdoo (Ed.), *Family ethnicity: Strength in diversity* (Newbury Park, CA: Sage), pp. 81–89.

Sullivan, H. S. (1953). *The interpersonal theory of psychiatry.* New York: Norton.

Tamura, E. H. (1994). *Americanization, acculturation, and ethnic identity: The Nisei generation in Hawaii.* Urbana: University of Illinois Press.

Tannen, D. (1990). *You just don't understand: Women and men in communication.* New York: Morrow.

Taylor, R. J. (1986). Receipt of support from family among Black Americans. *Journal of Marriage and the Family, 48,* 67–77.

Taylor, R. L. (1977). The Black worker in "post-industrial" society. In D. Y. Wilkinson and R. L. Taylor (Eds.), *The Black male in America: perspectives on his status in contemporary society* (Chicago: Nelson-Hall), pp. 280–308.

Taylor, R. L. & Arbuckle, G. (1995). Confucianism. *Journal of Asian Studies, 54,* 347–354.

Tharp, R. G., Meadow, A., Lennhoff, S. G., & Satterfield, D. (1968). Changes in marriage roles accompanying the acculturation of the Mexican-American woman. *Journal of Marriage and the Family, 30,* 404–412.

Thibaut, J. W. & Kelley, H. H. (1959). *The social psychology of groups.* New York: John Wiley.

Thompson, B. (1984). *Canonical correlation analysis: Uses and interpretation.* Newbury Park, CA: Sage.

Thornton, M. C. (1992). The quiet immigration: Foreign spouses of U. S. citizens. In M. P. Root (Ed.), *Racially mixed people in America* (Newbury Park, CA: Sage), pp. 64–76.

Tien, L. (1994). Southeast Asian American refugee women. In L. Comas-Diaz and B. Greene (Eds.), *Women of color: Integrating ethnic and gender identities in psychotherapy* (New York: Guilford), pp. 479–503.

Tinney, J. S. (1981). The religious experience of Black men. In L. E. Gary (Ed.), *Black men* (Beverly Hills, CA: Sage), pp. 269–276.

Triandis, H. C. (1990). Cross-cultural studies of individualism and collectivism. In J. J. Berman (Ed.), *Nebraska symposium on motivation 1989: Cross-cultural perspectives* (Lincoln: University of Nebraska Press), pp. 41–133.

Triandis, H. C., Hui, C. H., Albert, R. D., Leung, S., Lisansky, J., Diaz-Loving, R., Plascencia, L., Marin, G., Betancourt, H., & Loyola-Cintron, L. (1984). Individual models of social behavior. *Journal of Personality and Social Psychology, 46*, 1389–1404.

Triandis, H. C., Marin, G., Lisansky, J., & Betancourt, H. (1984). Simpatia as a cultural script of Hispanics. *Journal of Personality and Social Psychology, 47*, 1363–1375.

Triandis, H. C., McCusker, C., Betancourt, H., Iwao, S., Leung, K., Salazar, J. M., Setiadi, B., Sinha, J. B. P., Touzard, H., & Zaliski, Z. (1993). An emic-etic analysis of individualism and collectivism. *Journal of Cross-Cultural Psychology, 24*, 366–383.

Triandis, H. C., Weldon, D., & Feldman, J. (1972). *Black and White hardcore and middle class subjective cultures: A cross-validation.* Champaign: University of Illinois.

Tucker, M. B. & Mitchell-Kernan, C. M. (1990). New trends in Black American interracial marriage: The social structural context. *Journal of Marriage and the Family, 52*, 209–218.

Tucker, M. B. & Mitchell-Kernan, C. M. (1995). Social structure and psychological correlates of interethnic dating. *Journal of Social and Personal Relationships, 12*, 341–361.

Ullman, A. D. (1965). The framework. In A. D. Ullman (Ed.), *Sociocultural foundations of personality* (Boston: Houghton Mifflin), pp. 1–6.

Vasquez, M. J. T. (1984). Power and status of the Chicana: A social-psychological perspective. In J. L. Martinez, Jr. and R. H. Mendoza (Eds.), *Chicano psychology*, 2nd ed. (Orlando, FL: Academic Press), pp. 269–287.

Vasquez, M. J. T. (1994). Latinas. In L. Comas-Diaz and B. Greene (Eds.), *Women of color: Integrating ethnic and gender identities in psychotherapy* (New York: Guilford), pp. 114–138.

Wallace, M. (1979). *Black macho and the myth of the superwoman.* New York: Dial Press.

Wallis, W. D. (1935). Social history of the White man. In C. Murchison (Ed.), *A handbook of social psychology*, vol. 1 (New York: Russell & Russell), pp. 309–360.

Washington, J. R., Jr. (1970). *Marriage in Black and White.* Boston: Beacon.

Webster, Y. C. (1992). *The racialization of America.* New York: St. Martin's Press.

Wei, W. (1993). *The Asian American movement.* Philadelphia: Temple University Press.

References

West, C. (1993). *Race matters*. Boston: Beacon.

White, J. L. (1984). *The psychology of Blacks: An Afro-American perspective*. Englewood Cliffs, NJ: Prentice Hall.

White, J. L. & Parham, T. A. (1990). *The psychology of Blacks: An African-American perspective*. Englewood Cliffs, NJ: Prentice Hall.

Wiggins, J. S. (1979). A psychological taxonomy of trait-descriptive terms: The interpersonal domain. *Journal of Personality and Social Psychology, 37*, 395–412.

Wiggins, J. S. (1991). Agency and communion as conceptual coordinates for the understanding and measurement of interpersonal behavior. In W. M. Grove and D. Cicchetti (Eds.), *Thinking clearly about psychology*, vol. 2 (Minneapolis: University of Minnesota Press), pp. 89–113.

Wiggins, J. S. & Broughton, R. (1985). The Interpersonal Circle: A structural model for the integration of personality research. In R. Hogan & W. H. Jones (Eds.), *Perspectives in personality: A research annual*, (Greenwich, CT: JAI Press), pp. 1–47.

Wiggins, J. S. & Holzmuller, A. (1978). Psychological androgyny and interpersonal behavior. *Journal of Consulting and Clinical Psychology, 46*, 40–52.

Wilkinson, D. Y. (1977). The stigmatization process: The politicization of the Black male's identity. In D. Y. Wilkinson and R. L. Taylor (Eds.), *The Black male in America: Perspectives on his status in contemporary society* (Chicago: Nelson-Hall), pp. 145–158.

Wilkinson, D. Y. (1993). Family ethnicity in America. In H. P. McAdoo (Ed.), *Family ethnicity: Strength in diversity* (Newbury Park, CA: Sage), pp. 15–59.

Willems, E. (1975). *Latin American culture: An anthropological synthesis*. New York: Harper & Row.

Williams, C. W. (1991). *Black teenage mothers: Pregnancy and child rearing from their perspective*. Lexington, MA: Lexington Books.

Williams, N. (1990). *The Mexican American family: Tradition and change*. Dix Hills, NY: General Hall.

Willie, C. V. & Greenblatt, S. L. (1978). Four "classic" studies of power relationships in Black families: A review and look to the future. *Journal of Marriage and the Family, 40*, 691–694.

Wilson, C. C., III & Gutierrez, F. (1985). *Minorities and media: Diversity and the end of mass communication*. Beverly Hills, CA: Sage.

Wilson, W. J. (1980). *The declining significance of race: Blacks and changing American institutions*, 2nd ed. Chicago: University of Chicago Press.

Winstead, B. A. & Derlega, V. J. (1993). Gender and close relationships: An introduction. *Journal of Social Issues*, *49*, 1–9.

Wolf, F. M. (1986). *Meta-analysis: Quantitative methods for research synthesis*. Newbury Park, CA: Sage.

Wood, J. T. (1995). Feminist scholarship and the study of relationships. *Journal of Social and Personal Relationships*, *12*, 103–120.

Wood, J. T. & Duck, S. (1995). Off the beaten track: New shores for relationship research. In J. T. Wood and S. Duck (Eds.), *Under-studied relationships: Off the beaten track* (Thousand Oaks, CA: Sage), pp. 1–21.

Wyne, M. D., White, K. P., & Coop, R. H. (1974). *The Black self*. Englewood Cliffs, NJ: Prentice Hall.

Xiaohe, X. & Whyte, M. K. (1990). Love matches and arranged marriages: A Chinese replication. *Journal of Marriage and the Family*, *52*, 709–722.

Yu, A-B. & Yang, K-S. (1994). The nature of achievement motivation in collectivist societies. In U. Kim, H. C. Triandis, C. Kagitcibasi, S-C. Choi, and G. Yoon (Eds.), *Individualism and collectivism: Theory, methods, and applications* (Newbury Park, CA: Sage), pp. 239–250.

Zack, N. (1993). *Race and mixed race*. Philadelphia: Temple University Press.

Zapata, J. T. & Jaramillo, P. T. (1981). The Mexican American family: An Adlerian perspective. *Hispanic Journal of Behavioral Sciences*, *3*, 275–290.

Zavella, P. (1987). *Women's work and Chicano families: Cannery workers of the Santa Clara Valley*. Ithaca, NY: Cornell University Press.

Zeff, S. B. (1982). A cross-cultural study of Mexican American, Black American, and White American women at a large urban university. *Hispanic Journal of Behavioral Sciences*, *4*, 245–261.

Zinn, M. B. & Eitzen, D. S. (1987). *Diversity in American families*. New York: Harper & Row.

Zollar, A. C. (1985). *A member of the family: Strategies for Black family continuity*. Chicago: Nelson-Hall.